Essential Nursing Skills

For Mosby:

Senior Commissioning Editor: Ninette Premdas
Project Development Manager: Mairi McCubbin
Project Manager: Morven Dean
Designer: Judith Wright
Illustrations manager: Bruce Hogarth

Essential Nursing Skills

SECOND EDITION

Maggie Nicol
BSc(Hons) MSc PGDipEd RGN
Senior Lecturer, Clinical Skills

Carol Bavin
DipN(Lond) RCNT RGN RM
Lecturer

Shelagh Bedford-Turner
RGN BSc(Hons) MSc(Nursing) DipN(Cert Ed)
Lecturer

Patricia Cronin
BSc(Hons) MSc(Nursing) DipN(Lond) RGN
Senior Lecturer

Karen Rawlings-Anderson
BA(Hons) MSc(Nursing) DipN Ed RGN
Senior Lecturer

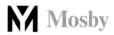

EDINBURGH LONDON NEW YORK OXFORD PHILADELPHIA ST LOUIS SYDNEY TORONTO 2003

MOSBY
An imprint of Elsevier Limited

First edition 2000
Second edition 2004
   Reprinted 2004

ISBN 0 7234 3307 0

British Library Cataloguing in Publication Data
A catalogue record for this book is available from the British Library

Library of Congress Cataloging in Publication Data
A catalog record for this book is available from the Library of Congress

Note
Medical knowledge is constantly changing. Standard safety precautions must be followed, but as new research and clinical experience broaden our knowledge, changes in treatment and drug therapy may become necessary or appropriate. Readers are advised to check the most current product information provided by the manufacturer of each drug to be administered to verify the recommended dose, the method and duration of administration, and contraindications. It is the responsibility of the practitioner, relying on experience and knowledge of the patient, to determine dosages and the best treatment for each individual patient. Neither the Publisher nor the authors assume any liability for any injury and/or damage to persons or property arising from this publication.

The Publisher

your source for books,
journals and multimedia
in the health sciences
www.elsevierhealth.com

Printed in China

Contents

Monitoring fluid balance; Application of a penile sheath; Observation of urine; Urinalysis; Midstream specimen of urine; Catheter specimen of urine; 24-hour urine collection; Urine specimen for cytology; Early morning specimen of urine; Female catheterisation; Male catheterisation; Catheter care; Emptying a catheter bag; Continuous bladder irrigation; Bladder washout; Catheter removal; Care of a stoma; Changing a stoma bag

Preface

Why this book?

As nurse teachers who teach clinical skills to undergraduate nursing students and newly qualified nurses, we wanted to write a book that detailed how to perform the skills and could serve as a reminder for the skills they had been taught but may not have had an opportunity to practise for several weeks, maybe months. The book is designed to be small enough to carry around, especially when in clinical practice. The practice of nursing is dynamic and rapidly changing. This second edition has been thoroughly updated to reflect new guidelines and nursing practices.

What is it?

This book deliberately focuses on the skills required by nurses caring for adult patients in a hospital setting, but the skills themselves can be adapted to any clinical setting. It is a manual of skills that are essential to nursing: a 'how-to-do-it' book. It is not a textbook and so does not include all the theory and rationale that underpins the various skills, but suggestions for further reading are provided at the end of each chapter. Most skills are accompanied by 'Points for Practice' **PFP** , a section that provides hints, suggestions or explanations to ensure successful performance of the skill.

The focus is on the practical aspects rather than why the skill is necessary. For example, insertion of a nasogastric tube explains how to select, measure and insert the tube; it does not discuss the reasons why such a tube may be necessary. This book is designed to complement nursing textbooks, not replace them.

How do I use it?

Each skill first describes preparation of the patient, the environment and the nurse, and the equipment needed. This is followed by a step-by-step description of the procedure, supported by illustrations, and additional information in the 'Points for Practice'. The care required following the skill is then described. *Essential Nursing Skills* is designed to act as a reminder for skills that you have been taught, and to enable you to prepare yourself for new skills. *As with all aspects of nursing, it is vital that a Registered Nurse supervises you until you have really mastered each skill and are competent to carry them out alone.*

Nursing practice is subject to many local policies and protocols and the reader is reminded to refer to them throughout. Local policies and protocols refer to specific aspects of nursing practice that may vary between hospitals and include: drug-checking procedures (e.g. intravenous drug therapy); which nurses are permitted to perform the skill (e.g. male catheterisation); which dressing should be used (e.g. care of an intravenous cannula); the way equipment should be cleaned (e.g. dressing trolley); and the disposal of clinical waste. Notes pages have been included to enable you to make a note of relevant local policies and procedures.

We hope that you will find this book interesting, enjoyable and a valuable resource to support and enhance your clinical practice.

London, 2003

Maggie Nicol
Carol Bavin
Shelagh Bedford-Turner
Patricia Cronin
Karen Rawlings-Anderson

1

Observation and monitoring

Preparation

Patient

- Explain the procedure, to gain consent and co-operation.
- The patient should be resting, either lying down or sitting. Allow time to rest after physical activity, emotional upset or smoking.

Equipment/Environment

- A watch with a second hand.
- Observation chart.

Nurse

- No special preparation is necessary unless required by the patient's condition, e.g. methicillin-resistant *Staphylococcus aureus* (MRSA).

Procedure

1. Choose a site to record the pulse. For most routine recordings the radial pulse is used **PFP1,2** (Figure 1.1).
2. Using your first and second fingers to feel the pulse, lightly but firmly compress the artery.
3. Count the number of beats for 1 minute. If the pulse is regular, it is sufficient to count for 30 seconds and double the result. If the pulse is irregular, count for a full minute.
4. In addition to the rate per minute, note the rhythm, i.e. whether it is regular or irregular, and the volume/strength of the pulse felt.

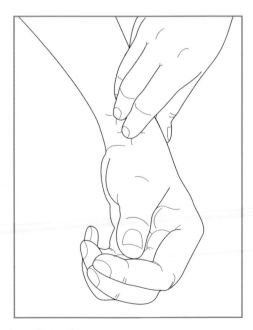

Figure 1.1 Taking the radial pulse

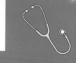

5. Note the colour of the patient's skin and mucous membranes (inside lower eyelid). Pallor may indicate anaemia, while a bluish colour indicates a lack of oxygen (cyanosis). In dark-skinned patients it is easier to detect this in the nail beds.

Post procedure

Patient

• Explain the results and discuss the reasons for any changes in care.

Nurse

• Record the findings and report any abnormalities.

Points for practice

1. The usual site for recording the pulse rate is at the wrist, where the radial pulse is easily felt.

2. Pulses may also be felt at other sites (see page 30) and these may be used to check tissue perfusion (e.g. following surgery to a limb) or in an emergency when the radial pulse would not be appropriate.

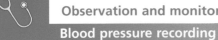

Preparation

Patient
- The patient should be resting in a bed, couch or chair, in a quiet location, with their legs uncrossed.
- The patient should not have had a meal, alcohol or caffeine or have smoked or exercised in the previous 30 minutes.

Equipment/Environment
- Sphygmomanometer with appropriate size cuff **PFP1,2**.
- Stethoscope.
- Alcohol-impregnated swabs.
- Observation chart.

Nurse
- The hands should be clean.
- No special preparation is necessary unless required by the patient's condition, e.g. MRSA.

Procedure

1. Assess the patient's knowledge of the procedure and explain as necessary.
2. Ensure the patient is resting in a comfortable position. If a comparison between lying and standing blood pressure is required, the 'lying' recording should be done first.
3. When applying the cuff, no clothing should be underneath it. If clothing constricts the arm, remove the arm from the sleeve **PFP3**.
4. Apply the cuff such that the centre of the 'bladder' is over the brachial artery, 2–3cm above the antecubital fossa **PFP4**.
5. The arm should be positioned so that the cuff is level with the heart and may be more comfortable resting on a pillow.
6. The sphygmomanometer should be placed on a firm surface, with the dial clearly visible.
7. Perform radial check to estimate systolic BP (PFPs). Locate the radial pulse. Squeeze the bulb slowly to inflate the cuff while still feeling the pulse. Observe the dial and note the level when the pulse can no longer be felt. Open the valve fully to quickly release the pressure in the cuff.
8. If using a communal stethoscope, clean the earpieces with an alcohol-impregnated swab. Curving the ends of the stethoscope slightly forward, place the earpieces in your ears. Check that the tubes are not twisted.
9. Check that the stethoscope is turned to the diaphragm side by tapping it with your finger.
10. Palpate the brachial artery, which is located on the medial aspect of the antecubital fossa (just to the side of the midline, on the side nearest to the patient) (Figure 1.2).

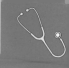

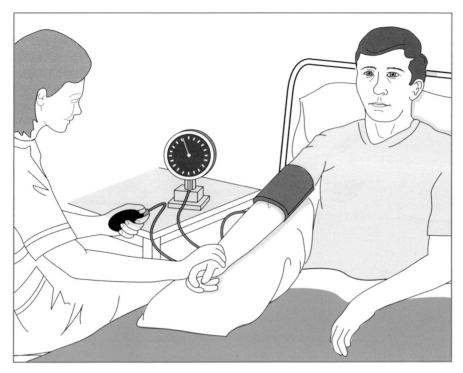

Figure 1.2 Radial check to estimate systolic BP

11. Place the diaphragm of the stethoscope over the artery, and hold it in place with your thumb while your fingers support the patient's elbow (Figure 1.3).
12. Position yourself so that the dial of the sphygmomanometer is clearly visible.
13. Ensure that the valve on the bulb is closed and inflate the cuff to 20–30mmHg above the level noted in step 7. Open the valve to allow the needle of the dial to drop **slowly** (2mm per second).
14. While observing the needle of the dial as it falls, listen for Korotkoff (thudding) sounds:
    • The **systolic** pressure is the level where these are first heard.
    • The **diastolic** pressure is the level where the sounds disappear.
15. Once the sounds have disappeared, open the valve fully, to completely deflate the cuff, and remove it from the patient's arm.
16. If a lying and standing BP is required, do not remove the cuff. Ask the patient to stand and then repeat steps 10–15 of the procedure PFP6,7 .

Post procedure

Patient

• Replace clothing and ensure the patient is comfortable.

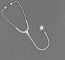
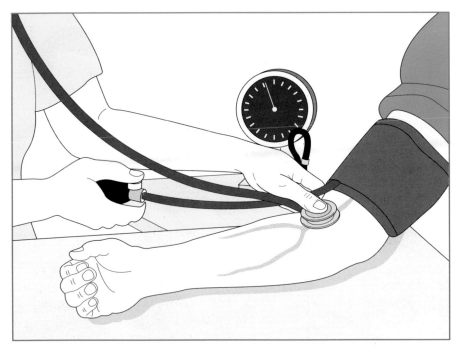

Figure 1.3 Stethoscope over the brachial artery

Equipment/Environment
- Replace equipment.
- Clean the earpieces of the stethoscope.

Nurse
- Chart the blood pressure accurately. Report any variation from previous recordings.

Points for practice

1. The sphygmomanometer may be an aneroid or a mercury type. These are used in exactly the same way except that a column of mercury, which must be placed in an upright position, is observed instead of a dial. Because mercury releases dangerous fumes if spilt, aneroid sphygmomanometers are replacing the mercury type.

2. The bladder inside the cuff must cover at least 80% of the circumference of the upper arm.

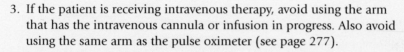

3. If the patient is receiving intravenous therapy, avoid using the arm that has the intravenous cannula or infusion in progress. Also avoid using the same arm as the pulse oximeter (see page 277).

4. If the patient is unable to lift their arm, tuck the patient's hand under your arm to support the arm while you position the cuff.

5. The radial check allows you to estimate the systolic blood pressure and avoid inflating the cuff unnecessarily high during step 13. This can be performed while palpating the brachial artery instead.

6. If recording lying and standing blood pressure, do not remove the cuff between recordings, keep it in the same position. The doctor may have requested that the patient is standing for at least 5 minutes before the standing blood pressure is recorded. Be aware that the patient may feel dizzy on getting out of bed (postural hypotension).

7. Electronic blood pressure recording machines are now often used. The cuff should be positioned in the same way as described in step 4, but no stethoscope is required because the machine provides a digital display of the systolic and diastolic pressures.

Preparation

Patient

- Explain the procedure, to gain consent and co-operation.
- Explain the need for bed rest while on the monitor **PFP1** .
- Ensure privacy.

Equipment/Environment

- Cardiac monitor with leads. This should have a maintenance sticker showing that it is safe to use.
- Disposable electrodes.
- Disposable razor or clippers (to remove chest hair).

Nurse

- No special preparation is necessary unless indicated by the patient's condition, e.g. MRSA.

Procedure

1. Place the cardiac monitor on a firm surface close to an electrical socket. Do not put anything on top of the monitor and keep the patient's drinks, etc., away from it.
2. Raise the bed to a safe working height.
3. Expose the patient's chest and examine the sites for the electrodes.
4. If chest is very hairy, shave a small patch at each site to allow good contact and adhesion of the electrodes.
5. Check the expiry date of the electrodes and ensure that they have not become dried out.
6. If the electrode has a small raised patch on the back, use this to roughen the skin slightly where the electrode will be placed. This improves adhesion and contact.
7. Remove the backing paper and taking care not to touch the gel in the middle, stick the electrodes firmly to the chest wall.
8. Connect the leads to the electrodes. This is usually by means of a small clip or press stud. The leads are labelled or colour coded and are connected as shown in Figure 1.4 **PFP2** .
9. Turn on the monitor and select lead II, which should produce the most positive (upright looking) display. If lead II does not produce a good display, try lead I or lead III. If necessary, adjust the 'gain' on the monitor to make the display larger and easier to see.
10. Set the alarms to safe parameters, according to the patient's condition.

Post procedure

Patient

- Explain/demonstrate what will happen if the patient moves or disturbs the electrodes (i.e. abnormal-looking pattern) to prevent unnecessary concern.

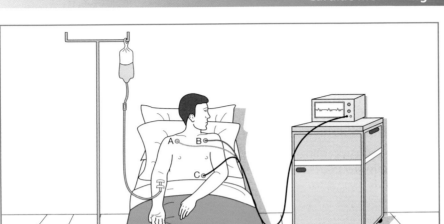

Figure 1.4 Cardiac monitoring

- Lower the bed.
- Replace clothing and ensure that the leads are not pulling on the electrodes.

Equipment/Environment

- Make sure all electrical cables are in good condition and are not under tension or trapped in any way, e.g. in bed rails, backrest, etc.
- Electrodes can usually remain in place for several days but may need replacing more frequently if the patient sweats a lot, if the electrode gel dries out, or if the patient's skin shows signs of sensitivity.

Nurse

- Note the rhythm shown on the monitor and if the monitor has the facility, take a printout, it is a good idea to do this at the beginning of each shift. Observe for any arrhythmias and report as appropriate.

Points for practice

1. In the acute situation, most patients with cardiac monitors are required to rest in bed. However, patients undergoing investigations for cardiac rhythm abnormalities may have a 24-hour tape or ambulatory monitoring system (telemetry), in which case they may move around but should always inform the nurses of their whereabouts.

2. The leads are referred to as limb leads even though they are attached to the chest. This is because they represent that area of the body, i.e. right arm, left arm and left leg.

Preparation

Patient

- Explain the procedure, to gain consent and co-operation.
- Explain the need to lie still during this procedure.
- Ensure privacy.

Equipment/Environment

- A 12-lead electrocardiography (ECG) machine and leads, and paper for printout.
- Disposable electrodes for limb and chest leads (usually adhesive with clips or press studs).

Nurse

- No special preparation is necessary unless indicated by the patient's condition, e.g. MRSA.

Procedure

1. Ask/assist the patient to lie in a recumbent or semi-recumbent position.
2. Raise the bed to a safe working height.
3. Expose the patient's ankles, wrists and chest area.
4. Apply the electrodes to the patient's ankles and wrists as shown in Figure 1.5A **PFP1**.
5. Apply the electrodes to the chest wall as shown in Figure 1.5B. If necessary, shave the area to ensure good contact/adhesion.
6. Connect the ECG leads to the electrodes as labelled or colour coded.
7. Ask the patient to lie still.
8. Press 'start' on the ECG machine. All 12 leads will print out on one page. Add the patient's name, ward and hospital number to the printout **PFP2**.

Post procedure

Patient

- Remove the electrodes and wipe away any traces of gel.
- Lower the bed to a safe level.
- Ensure the patient is comfortable.

Equipment/Environment

- Leave the ECG machine clean, tidy and stocked ready for the next user. Do not tie the leads together as this may damage them.

Nurse

- File the ECG printout in the patient's notes.
- Inform the requesting doctor/nurse that the ECG is available.

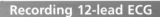

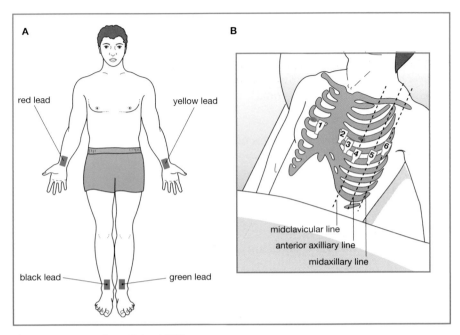

Figure 1.5 Recording 12-lead ECG
A = Position of limb leads
B = Position of chest leads

Points for practice

1. If the patient is an amputee, apply the electrode to the stump.

2. It is usual to note whether the patient has chest pain or is pain free at the time of the ECG recording.

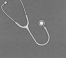

Preparation

Patient

- Explain the need for frequent observations, even throughout the night. Observations must be continued and sleeping patients must be woken to check that they are not in a coma.

Equipment/Environment

- A small, bright torch for pupil reactions.
- Sphygmomanometer and stethoscope and thermometer.
- Glasgow Coma Scale chart (see page 16).
- If the patient is confused and restless, bed rails padded with pillows may be needed. The bed should be at its lowest level.

Nurse

- No special preparation is necessary unless required by the patient's condition, e.g. MRSA.

Procedure

The Glasgow Coma Scale (page 16) assesses the level of consciousness by monitoring the patient's ability in eye opening, motor response and verbal response. Each activity is scored according to the stimulus needed to elicit a response from the patient. The worst total score is 3 and the best 15. Any reduction in the score is a sign that the patient's consciousness level is deteriorating and should be reported immediately. A patient with a score of 8 or less will be in a deep coma.

Three levels of stimuli are usually adopted: auditory (a question, a command or a noise like hand clapping); tactile (touch); and painful stimuli, which are considered the most powerful.

Assessment of eye opening

Eye opening demonstrates that the arousal mechanisms in the brain are functioning and the scoring system is used as follows:

4 = patients who are conscious, who sense your approach and open their eyes spontaneously or patients who are asleep but open their eyes in response to a verbal stimulus or light touch.
3 = patients who open their eyes in response to a verbal stimulus.
2 = patients who open their eyes only in response to a painful stimulus. The normal response to pain is to draw away from the stimulus by moving the limb or trying to push the nurse's hand away. Pain response can be tested either centrally (by trapezium squeeze, pinching and twisting the muscle where the head meets the shoulder) or peripherally (pressing firmly on the side of the finger or the earlobes). Other methods (e.g. rubbing the sternum or pressing on nail beds) are no longer recommended. Although it seems cruel to inflict pain, it is important to assess the response to pain if the patient does not react to less unpleasant stimuli.
1 = no eye opening in response to verbal or painful stimuli.

Patients may not be able to open their eyes if there is damage to the occulo-motor nerve, which is responsible for movement of the eyelid. If the patient is unable to open their eyes due to swelling, trauma or an eye dressing, this is indicated using the letter 'C'. If unable to open their eyes due to medication (e.g. paralysing agents) this is indicated using the letter 'P'.

Verbal response

This assesses whether patients are aware of themselves and their environment. If the patient has a tracheostomy or an endotracheal tube, the letter 'T' can be used to indicate this. The score is used as follows.

5 = the patient is orientated, i.e. able to tell the nurse who they are, where they are, what day, date, month and year it is, and why they are where they are.
4 = the patient is able to hold a conversation but not able to answer specific questions (i.e. confused and not orientated).
3 = the patient can speak but does so randomly and makes verbal responses such as swearing or shouting.
2 = speech is incomprehensible and the nurse may have to use painful stimuli to get a response.
1 = the patient does not respond to verbal and painful stimuli.

If the patient is unable to speak (dysphasia) it may be due to damage to speech centres in the brain. There are two types: receptive dysphasia (when patients cannot understand the spoken word) and expressive dysphasia (when they are unable to reply with the correct words). In both cases, a score of 1 is given and the dysphasia is noted by using the letter 'D'.

Motor response

When assessing motor response, scores are allocated as follows.

6 = obeying commands (the best response). Instructions may include 'lift your arms' or 'squeeze my hands'.
5 = localising to pain, which means that the patient's brain is receiving sensory information regarding the process of feeling pain. When assessing for this response a central pain stimulus (see 'assessment of eye opening' above) is used. Patients will usually respond by trying purposefully to remove the source of the pain. An arm is used to test this because leg responses are less reliable and can be a spinal reflex rather than a brain response. If the patient cannot be assessed due to presence of fractures, this can be documented using the symbol '#'. The best (and safest) stimulus to assess this response is the trapezium squeeze (see 'assessment of eye opening' above).
4 = the patient withdraws from pain or moves towards the source of the pain but does not attempt to remove it.
3 = abnormal flexion, which is an abnormal response such as wrist rotation and arm or elbow flexion. This usually indicates that the nerve pathways are not functioning normally and in some cases is a sign of deterioration and a poor prognosis.

13

2 = the patient extends to pain and may rotate the arm inwards or extend or straighten the arm at the elbow. This indicates damage to the brain stem and the prognosis for the patient is very poor.

1 = no response to pain. Patients who are deemed to be 'brain dead' will score 1.

Pupil response

Raised intracranial pressure causes changes in the size of the pupils and their response to light. Assessment of the pupils (Figure 1.6) assesses the function of the optic nerve, which causes a reaction to light being shone in the eye, and the occulomotor nerve, which constricts the pupil. A poor reaction in either of these assessments indicates compression of the nerves. When undertaking assessment of the pupils, dim the light in the room and hold the eyelid open. Before you shine the light in the patient's eye observe the following.

- The resting size of both pupils. The average size if 2–5mm but it varies according to the time of the day.
- See if both pupils are equal in size – inequality can be a serious sign of raised intracranial pressure.
- Look at the shape of the pupils – they are normally round. Different shapes can indicate damage to the brain.

Bringing the light of the pen torch in from the side of the eye, observe:

- the reaction of each pupil to light
- the intensity of the reaction, i.e. whether it is brisk, sluggish or absent.

It is also important to note if the patient has a pre-existing abnormality or irregularity of the eye/s, for example cataracts, which will affect the response. In addition it is important to note the drugs or medications the patients may have had. Some cause dilation (e.g. atropine) whilst others (opiates e.g. morphine) cause constriction.

Vital signs

These are not part of the Glasgow Coma Scale itself but because of their importance, they are usually included on the same chart (Figure 1.7).

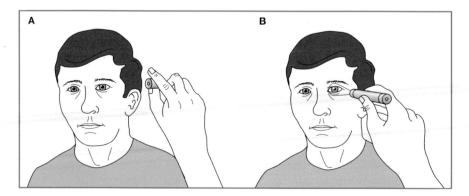

Figure 1.6 Assessment of pupil response and size

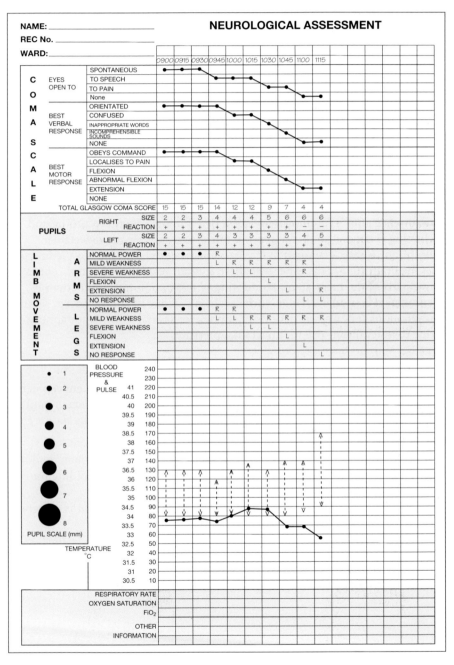

NEUROLOGICAL ASSESSMENT

NAME: _____

REC No. _____

WARD: _____

Figure 1.7 Neurological assessment of a patient with a right hemisphere space-occupying lesion.

- **Temperature** – alterations in patients' temperature may be due to damage of the thermoregulation centre of the brain. A rise in body temperature increases the demand for oxygen by the brain cells, which may already be compromised due to damage. It is desirable to keep the body temperature within normal limits, where possible. This may require antipyretic agents such as paracetamol or active measures such as fan therapy (see page 24).
- **Pulse rate and blood pressure** – in patients with raised intracranial pressure the blood pressure rises and pulse rate falls. As the brain becomes hypoxic and ischaemic, the body responds by attempting to increase the arterial blood pressure in order to get oxygen to it. As a result there is a need for more blood in each contraction of the heart. This results in a slowing of the heart rate (bradycardia). Respiration rate also decreases and a change in the respiratory pattern occurs. This is known as 'Cushing's reflex' and is a very late occurrence after level of consciousness deteriorates. Careful recording and charting is needed so that a trend in this direction is clearly detectable.
- **Respiration rate** – changes in respiration are a good indicator of the function of the brain stem. This is because there are four respiratory control centres in two parts of the brain stem. Monitoring of respiration rate and pattern is essential as a sudden change, such as Cheyne–Stoke breathing (deep, sighing respirations followed by periods of apnoea for several seconds) or apnoea, is due to a significant rise in intracranial pressure.

Limb movement

In addition to motor response assessment, assessing limb movement can detect weaknesses of one side of the body or limbs. Assessing limb movement and motor power gives an indication of the extent of the damage to the motor cortex that controls motor movement and is graded as follows.

- **Normal power** – the nurse applies resistance to any joint movement and this can be matched by the patient, e.g. pulling or pushing whilst holding the hands.
- **Mild weakness** – the patient is able to counter the resistance but is overcome easily.
- **Severe weakness** – the patient is able to move the limb but not against resistance.
- **Flexion, extension or no response** – there is flexion, extension or no movement in response to central or peripheral painful stimuli.

Preparation

Patient

- Protecting the patient from injury is of primary concern.
- Maintain privacy and dignity where possible **PFP1**.

Equipment/Environment

- Ensure patient safety. This may entail clearing the environment or, on rare occasions, moving the patient from danger.

Nurse

- Maintain own safety.

Procedure

When the patient has a seizure **PFP2**, the first phase (the tonic phase) is associated with rigidity of limbs and breath holding. This phase may be brief. In the second phase (clonic phase), there is rhythmical jerking of arms and legs. Characteristically the jerks are unilateral, initially close together and then decreasing in frequency. This phase is followed by a period of deep sleep, when the patient is usually unrousable and their body is limp.

1. Protect the patient from injury but do not attempt to restrain their limbs.
2. Use pillows as necessary to pad hard surfaces, and remove non-essential furniture and equipment.
3. Observe the patient continuously, noting the following:
   - Duration of each phase of the seizure, including the recovery time (i.e. when able to resume normal activities).
   - Limbs involved.
   - Whether movement is localised or general.
   - Whether the jaw is clenched **PFP3**.
   - Whether the patient is frothing at the mouth (saliva).
   - Whether the patient has been incontinent of urine or faeces.
   - Breathing pattern – this will change. Patients are likely to hold their breath and may become cyanosed or just pale. Loud breathing sounds may indicate the end of the seizure. (The breathing reverts spontaneously and oxygen is not usually required.)
4. During the period of deep sleep following the clonic phase, the patient should be left in the recovery position to maintain an airway (see page 42) and should not be disturbed, allowing the patient to recover in their own time. It can last up to 30 minutes.
5. It is now safe to put your fingers in the patient's mouth to remove food or dentures if necessary.
6. If seizures occur in rapid succession this is called status epilepticus and requires urgent medical intervention.

Post procedure

Patient

- Reassure patient by being calm and explaining what has happened.
- Ask patient whether there was any warning of the seizure (aura) and whether it can be described, e.g. a smell or taste.

Equipment/Environment

- Ensure patient comfort by offering a wash, change of clothing, etc., as necessary.

Nurse

- All seizures must be documented and reported.
- If there is no previous history, the doctor must be informed.

Points for practice

1. If the seizure occurs in a public place, encourage bystanders to disperse to prevent the patient feeling crowded and possibly embarrassed.

2. The term 'fitting' refers to a patient suffering from a seizure with tonic and clonic phases. This was formerly called a grand mal fit.

3. During the tonic phase of the seizure, the patient will clench their jaw and may bite their tongue. Nothing should be inserted into the mouth to try and prevent this.

Preparation

Patient

- Explain procedure, to gain consent and co-operation.
- Assess patient regarding suitable site for temperature recording (PFP1,2).
- Patient should not have had a hot drink, smoked a cigarette or exercised within the previous 15 minutes.

Equipment/Environment

- Disposable chemical thermometer, e.g. TempaDot (PFP3,4).
- Observation chart.

Nurse

- Hands must be clean.

Procedure

Oral

1. Ask the patient to open their mouth, and gently insert the thermometer under their tongue, next to the frenulum (PFP1). This is adjacent to a large artery (sublingual artery), so the temperature will be close to core temperature (Figure 1.8A).
2. Ask the patient to close their lips, but not their teeth, around the thermometer, to prevent cool air circulating in the mouth.
3. Leave in position for the recommended length of time (usually 1 minute).
4. Remove the thermometer, taking care not to touch the part that has been in the patient's mouth. In accordance with the manufacturer's instructions, read the temperature by noting the way that the dots have changed colour (see Figure 1.8C).

Axilla

1. Ask/assist the patient to expose their axilla. For an accurate recording, the axilla must be dry.
2. With the dots facing the chest wall, position the thermometer vertically between the arm and the chest wall and ask/assist the patient to keep their arm close against the chest to ensure good contact with the skin (see Figure 1.8B).
3. Leave in position for the recommended length of time (usually 3 minutes).
4. In accordance with the manufacturer's instructions, read the temperature by noting the way that the dots have changed colour (see Figure 1.8C).

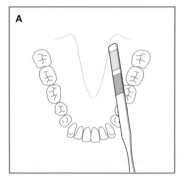
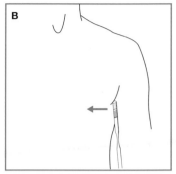
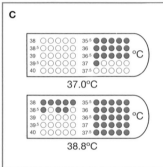

Figure 1.8 Disposable chemical thermometer
  A = Positioning the thermometer for oral use
  B = Positioning the thermometer for axillary use
  C = Reading the thermometer

Post procedure

Patient

- Ensure patient comfort.
- Answer any questions regarding the recording.

Equipment/Environment

- Dispose of the thermometer into the clinical waste bag.

Nurse

- Chart temperature recording.
- Report any abnormality.

Points for practice

1. If the patient is unconscious, confused, prone to seizures, has mouth sores or has undergone oral surgery, the oral site should not be used for temperature measurement.

2. The rectal site is no longer recommended except when an electronic probe is being used.

3. Mercury thermometers are no longer widely used as there are risks of breakage. If a mercury thermometer is used, it must be cleaned before and after use and the mercury must be shaken down to the bottom of the scale before use.

4. Electronic oral and tympanic thermometers are increasingly being used (see page 22).

Oral

Electronic oral thermometers are increasingly being used in hospitals. They are efficient, quick and easy to use, with an audible signal indicating when the maximum temperature has been reached. The probe, covered by a disposable plastic cover, is placed under the tongue in the same way as a disposable thermometer (Figure 1.9A). Each cover is for use by one patient only and is usually kept clean and dry on the patient's locker between uses. It is discarded when the patient is discharged from the ward.

Tympanic

Some electronic thermometers are designed to measure the temperature by inserting a probe into the outer ear, adjacent to (but not touching) the tympanic membrane (Figure 1.9B). An infrared light detects heat radiated from the tympanic membrane and provides a digital reading. This usually takes only a few seconds and an audible signal indicates when the reading is complete. This provides a more accurate measure of body core temperature as it is close to the carotid artery. A special cover is used for each patient to prevent cross-infection. The patient may need more explanation than usual because, although most people will have had their temperature recorded at some point, they may be surprised to find you approaching their ear! It is a simple technique but the following may lead to an inaccurate reading: wax in the ear; a cracked or dirty lens; poor fitting in the ear; and if the patient has been recently lying on the ear that is used (Jevon 2001).

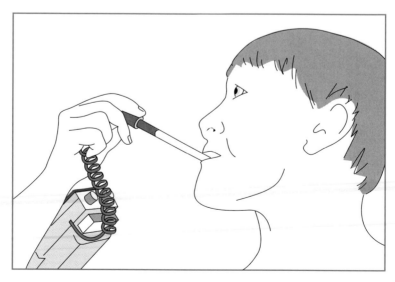

Figure 1.9 A = Oral electronic thermometer

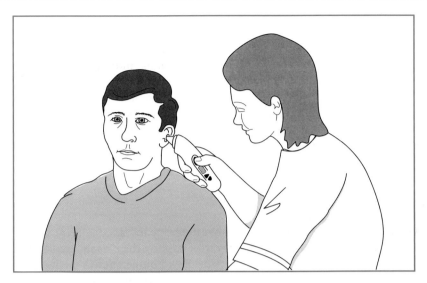

Figure 1.9 B = Tympanic membrane thermometer

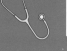
Tepid sponging

Tepid sponging is designed to reduce the patient's temperature. The skin is cooled by applying tepid water with a sponge or flannel to a whole limb or extensive area of the body and then allowing it to evaporate, taking heat with it. With even a slightly raised temperature, this can make the patient feel much refreshed. It is important to maintain dignity and privacy throughout this procedure. Tepid rather than cold water is used, as cold water would cause peripheral vasoconstriction, allowing less blood near the surface to be cooled. Cold water might also induce shivering, which may cause the temperature to rise rather than fall.

Fan therapy

Cooling the air around the patient so that the body loses more heat through radiation from the skin is an effective way of cooling the person. However, it is important that the fan is carefully placed to avoid blowing onto the face of the patient as this can cause drying of the cornea of the eyes, leading to ulceration. The fan should be an oscillating type so that cooling is gentle and covers all areas of the body.

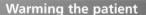

Patients, particularly the elderly, are often cold and may be suffering from hypothermia (a temperature of less than 35°C) on admission to hospital. This may be due to a lack of heating at home, exposure following an accident of some kind, or they may have been lying undiscovered for a period of time. It can also occur following lengthy surgery despite the use of warming methods during the operation. Warm air systems, which blow warm air through a disposable blanket onto the patient's body, are used to warm patients. A space blanket is made of thin, foil-type material that is designed to reflect back heat to prevent it being lost from the body. These are used in outdoor activities but are seen less often in the hospital setting. If the patient is receiving intravenous fluids or a blood transfusion, these can be warmed using a blood warmer (see page 94). If the patient is able to take oral fluids, hot drinks and soup are very effective. Humans lose a great deal of heat through their heads, so covering the head with a scarf or hat is beneficial. If the hypothermia is severe (temperature less than 32°C), internal warming methods, such as warm gastric or peritoneal lavage and warmed intravenous fluids, may be necessary.

Preparation

Patient

- Encourage the patient to empty their bladder.
- Weigh the patient on the same scales, at the same time each day/week, and in similar clothing.

Equipment/Environment

- The scales must be on a level surface.
- Use the same scales for regular weighing.
- Ensure the pointer is at zero or weights are to the left, at zero.

Nurse

- An apron should be worn if the patient requires assistance.

Procedure

1. Position the scales for easy access and apply the brakes.
2. Ask/assist the patient to sit on the scales or stand on the platform. If electronic scales are being used, plug them into the mains before the patient sits down.
3. If sitting, ensure that the patient's feet are off the floor.
4. Ask the patient to remain still, and note the reading.
5. If the scales are manual, check the patient's previous weight to determine the approximate position and move the heavier weight bar (kilograms) to the right until the two pivotal arrows swing (e.g. if the previous weight was 73kg, move the heavier bar to 70kg). If the bar is moved too far, the weight will sink and stop swinging. Adjust the lighter weight bar so that the arrows are exactly level and free floating.
6. Note the reading by adding the position of the heavier bar (e.g. 70kg) to that of the lighter bar (e.g. 3.5kg; total equals 73.5kg).
7. If the weight is very different from a recent previous weight, check it again and, if confirmed, report it.

Post procedure

Patient

- Assist the patient back to the bed/chair as necessary.

Equipment/Environment

- Return the scales to their storage place and clean if necessary.

Nurse

- Document weight and report any unexpected loss or gain.

Preparation

Patient

- Explain the procedure, to gain consent and co-operation.
- Ensure the patient's hands are clean. Do not use alcohol wipes **PFP1**.
- Ask the patient to choose the finger to be used for the procedure.

Equipment/Environment

- Glucose meter.
- Finger-pricking device or lancet.
- Gauze swab/cotton-wool ball, according to local policy.
- Blood glucose testing strips.

Nurse

- Wash and dry hands thoroughly.
- Put on gloves.

Procedure

1. Ensure all equipment is within easy reach and the patient is comfortable.
2. If necessary, assist the patient with washing and drying of the finger/hand.
3. Use new lancets and platforms (if finger-pricking device used) for each test **PFP2**.
4. Check the expiry date of the testing strips and prepare the glucose meter and insert the testing strip according to the manufacturer's instructions **PFP3**.
5. Using the appropriate device, prick the side of the patient's fingertip, avoiding the thumbs, index and little fingers where possible **PFP4**.
6. Allow a drop of blood to fall onto the testing strip – do not smear **PFP5**.
7. Ask the patient to press on the site, using the gauze swab/cotton-wool ball, to stem bleeding and reduce the risk of bruising.
8. Wait for the meter to provide a digital display of the result **PFP6**.

Post procedure

Patient

- Ensure the patient is comfortable.
- Ensure bleeding has stopped.

Equipment/Environment

- Dispose of all sharps and contaminated waste in the appropriate containers.
- Return equipment as appropriate.

Nurse

- Remove gloves and wash hands.
- Document the result and report any abnormalities.

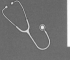

Points for practice

1. The patient's hands should be clean. If there is any possibility that there may have been contact with substances such as fruit juice, the finger should be wiped with a wet tissue and then a dry tissue before pricking. An alcohol swab should not be used as this may give a false reading.

2. Where possible use a finger-pricking device, as it is more likely to ensure a good blood flow and is less painful. Before pricking the patient's finger, hold the hand downwards to encourage blood flow, and make a light tourniquet with your hand around the finger to ensure sufficient blood is present in the tip of the finger. Avoid 'milking' blood into the finger as the local blood composition may be disturbed by intermingling with tissue fluid. Taking time to encourage blood flow before pricking the finger will reduce the need for pricking again, which can be distressing for the patient.

3. Preparation of the glucose meter usually involves checking that it has been calibrated for the particular batch of testing strips that are being used.

4. Blood glucose monitoring can be painful for the patient, especially if performed several times a day. Non-invasive methods of measuring blood glucose levels (e.g. Glucowatch™) are currently being developed.

5. The drop of blood should fall onto the strip rather than be 'wiped on', as this may lead to an inaccurate result.

6. With some glucose meters, the strip is inserted into the meter after the blood is dropped onto it. Follow the manufacturer's instructions regarding timing and wiping prior to insertion into the machine.

Preparation

Patient

- Explain procedure, to gain consent and co-operation.
- Explain the need for frequent observations **PFP1**.

Equipment/Environment

- Screening the bed is not usually necessary but ensure dignity and privacy is maintained.

Nurse

- Hands must be clean and dry.

Procedure

Assess the following:

1. Movement – ask the patient to move the toes/fingers of the affected area of the limb.
2. Sensation – without letting the patient see which toes/fingers you are touching, touch the toes/fingers randomly and ask the patient to tell you which one you are touching **PFP2**.
3. Pain/swelling – if the patient complains of pain or the toes/fingers are swollen, check the bandage, splint or plaster cast for tightness.
4. Temperature – the fingers/toes should be warm to touch.
5. Colour – the skin should be pink, indicating adequate perfusion. If the patient has dark skin, observe the nail beds.
6. Pulse – it may be possible to locate a pulse, particularly in the feet. Once located, this may be marked to make it easier for subsequent checking (Figure 1.10) **PFP3**.
7. Bandage/dressing/splint/plaster cast – check for bleeding and that the bandage/dressing, etc., is not too tight, causing constriction of the blood supply to the limb.

Post procedure

Patient

- Elevation of the affected limb will help prevent swelling.
- The elevated limb must be well supported.

Equipment/Environment

- Exposed extremities may be kept warm by using a loose-fitting sock or piece of tubular bandage.

Nurse

- Wash hands.

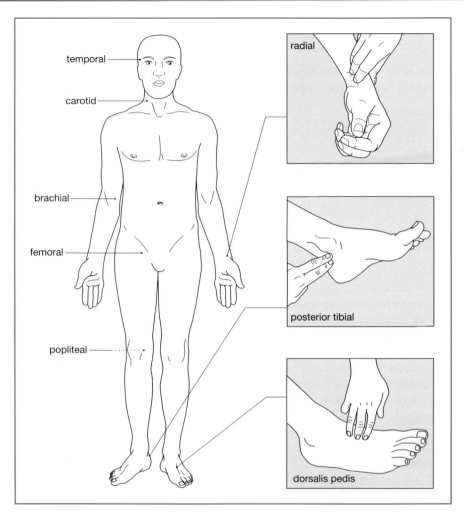

Figure 1.10 Peripheral pulses

Points for practice

1. These observations are made following injury or surgery to a limb. The limb may be bandaged, splinted or encased in plaster of Paris.

2. It is important to see all the fingers/toes move, particularly as little toes can be covered. Each digit has a separate nerve supply, which may be damaged or compressed.

3. If recording 'pulse not felt', take care that it not confused with 'pulse not able to be located' due to the bandage/splint, etc.

Principles

Pain is sometimes considered to be the fifth vital sign (after temperature, pulse, respirations & BP), which indicates the level of importance that should be placed on assessing and managing pain (Lynch 2001). This is because pain can have harmful physiological, psychological and emotional effects. Pain is a complex phenomenon and its successful management has always presented a challenge. There have been significant advances in the management of pain with the development of acute and chronic pain services, and improved techniques for administering analgesia, including patient-controlled analgesia (PCA) and epidural analgesia. Effective pain management depends on good interprofessional team working, and the nurse's role is central in ensuring that the patient's pain is assessed, treatment regimens are implemented and their effectiveness evaluated. This is a continuous process and it is suggested here that there are three key areas for consideration in the assessment of pain.

1. Who should assess the patient's pain?

Pain is largely a subjective experience and so patients themselves are best placed to assess their own pain accurately. Observation by others involves interpretation of what the patient is feeling and therefore can be unreliable. It is vital that nurses accept the patients' estimation of their pain even if it is not accompanied by the usual behaviours (e.g. grimacing, adopting a foetal position, groaning) or alteration to vital signs, e.g. raised pulse. Vital signs can be unreliable as a measure of a person's pain. The way in which different patients respond to pain can be attributed to a multitude of variables such as age, culture, type of pain, and duration. Observation and vital sign measurement should only be relied upon when the patient is unable to communicate. Assessment of pain is an important aspect of the nurse's role that requires a number of skills including observation, interpretation and communication skills.

2. When should the patient's pain be assessed?

The frequency of pain assessment is dependent on the individual circumstances. Factors to be considered when determining frequency include:

- The severity of the pain. Pain assessment is often carried out when the patient is resting but a better indicator of the efficacy of analgesia may be achieved by asking the patient to cough, move, take a deep breath.
- Frequency should be increased if pain is poorly controlled or treatment regimens are changing.
- Regular pain assessment is important in the post-operative period. Patients with patient-controlled analgesia (PCA) should be assessed each time other vital signs are recorded. In patients with epidural analgesia, the sensory block should be checked approximately 20 minutes after the administration of the analgesic.

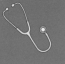
3. What should be assessed?

Initial assessment of a patient's pain should include:

- **The location, duration, intensity and characteristics of the pain**
Defining the nature of a patient's pain is important, as different types of pain
will be treated differently. The nurse should establish whether the pain is
localised to a particular part of the body or whether it is more generalised. The
patient should be asked to describe whether the pain is 'sharp', 'dull', 'intermittent' or 'continuous', and to indicate how long they have had it. The patient's
perception of the pain is important and this should be assessed in terms of
whether it is 'tolerable', 'unbearable', etc.
- **The underlying condition**
The underlying diagnosis or cause of a patient's pain is central to determining
whether the subsequent treatment is curative or palliative. For example, acute
pain is often an indicator of disease or injury, which, following treatment can
be resolved. Conversely, pain may indicate a worsening of the patient's condition but the overall goal of treatment may be palliative and focus on relieving
the symptoms.
- **Is the pain acute, chronic or acute on chronic?**
It is important to establish whether the patient's pain is acute, chronic or acute
on chronic, as this may influence the choice of treatment. For example, pharmacological intervention is the mainstay of acute pain management whereas
chronic pain management often demands a range of treatment options including pharmacological and non-pharmacological regimens.
- **Any medical/nursing treatment being given**
It is important to review any treatment currently being received by the patient
in order to determine its effectiveness. Furthermore, current treatment may be
an important indicator as to the efficacy of any proposed treatments.
- **Precipitating or exacerbating factors, e.g. mobility/immobility, time of day,
eating/drinking**
Determining factors that precipitate or exacerbate the pain facilitates diagnosis
and also aids with identification of the goals of care. For example, if a patient
develops pain when undertaking a particular activity, the goal of care may be
twofold. The patient may be encouraged to either avoid the activity or may
undertake a programme that concentrates on maximising their coping potential
in that situation. Time of day may also be significant; some patients report
higher levels of pain at night.
- **Related symptoms, e.g. nausea, vomiting, breathlessness or sleeplessness**
Related symptoms such as nausea and vomiting are often significant in aiding
diagnosis but are also important in that they can cause the patient such distress
as to interfere with their ability to cope with pain. A score to indicate the level
of nausea and vomiting is often used with patients receiving PCA. This should
be assessed and recorded with other vital signs. Pain that causes sleeplessness
significantly reduces the patient's ability to tolerate it.

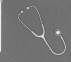

- **Coping strategies used by the patient – pharmacological and non-pharmacological**

When determining the plan of care for a patient in pain, it is important to include any coping strategies the patient may have developed. Medication used by the patient may indicate what 'works' and may subsequently minimise the risk of prescribing treatments which 'do not work'. Non-pharmacological coping strategies (such as use of heat pads or massage) should, whenever possible, be included in the overall plan of care. This will enhance the patient's perception of being involved in their plan of care.

- **Meaning or significance of the pain for the patient**

The patient's perception of the significance of their pain is extremely important. Pain creates fear, anxiety and a sense of loss of control. Fear of death is common. It is essential, therefore, for the nurse to establish how patients perceive their pain.

Self-report pain assessment tools

Initial and ongoing assessment may be undertaken using a Self-Reporting Pain Assessment Tool, the most common of which are:

- **Visual Analogue Scale**

The Visual Analogue Scale uses a 10cm line with one end-point indicating 'No Pain' and the other indicating 'Worst Pain Imaginable' (Figure 1.11). The patient indicates the point on the line that best represents their pain. Some scales include words at set intervals, e.g. 'slight', 'moderate', 'severe'.

- **Verbal Numerical Rating Scale**

The Verbal Numerical Rating Scale is similar to the Visual Analogue Scale. Using a scale in which 0 is 'no pain' and 10 is 'worst imaginable pain'; patients are asked to indicate the number that best represents their pain.

- **Categorical Rating Scale**

These scales ask the patient to consider a series of words which best describes the pain, e.g. 'none', 'mild', 'moderate', 'severe', 'very severe' and 'worst pain imaginable'.

Any of the above scales may be complemented by the use of a body outline that gives a good indication of pain sites. Providing the patient is able to understand the tool there are a number of advantages to using such scales:

- They can be used alone or in conjunction with other pain assessment.
- They are simple to use.
- They provide a clear picture of pain intensity.
- Regular use provides evidence of the efficacy of treatment regimens and indicates an improvement or worsening of the patient's pain experience.

It is vital that nurses regard pain assessment as a priority. Unless pain is assessed regularly and effectively, patients will continue to suffer unnecessarily. Effective pain assessment is a fundamental part of nursing care and accountability for the accuracy of pain assessment lies firmly within the domain of nursing.

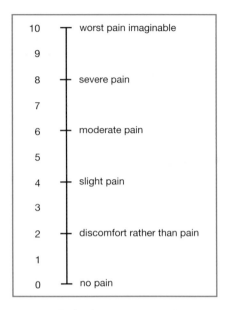

Figure 1.11 Visual analogue scale (with numeric values)

PATIENT-CONTROLLED ANALGESIA (PCA)

Principles

Patient-controlled analgesia (PCA) has become a popular method of managing post-operative pain since the early 1990s. However, today its use is not confined to post-operative pain management, it has been found to be useful in patients with burns, myocardial infarction, bone marrow transplantation and sickle cell crisis. It can also be useful with patients who are terminally ill. PCA facilitates active involvement of patients in the management of their pain. Through the use of a syringe driver and a timing device, PCA allows patients to self-administer small doses of an analgesic whenever they feel pain. It has several advantages over intermittent intramuscular or subcutaneous administration of analgesics on an 'as required' basis:

1. PCA gives the patient a sense of control and there is no questioning of the validity of the pain.
2. It enables analgesia requirement to be individualised to a sufficiently high plasma concentration level and stable plasma concentration levels to be maintained thereafter. This prevents the peaks and troughs associated with intermittent injection.
3. Unlike the conventional system of intermittent injection, there is no delay between the request for analgesia and the provision of pain relief.
4. It saves nurses' time.

   PCA is usually administered intravenously (although epidural and subcutaneous infusions are also possible) via a syringe driver and timing

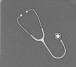

device. The patient activates the system by pressing a button that releases a small dose of the analgesic into the circulation. There is a 'lock-out' device that prevents further doses being delivered with a specified time interval (usually between 5 and 20 minutes depending on the drug and the dosage). The use of the lock-out device reduces the risk of overdose. Morphine is the most common opiate used and a dose of 1mg at 10-minute intervals will usually provide effective pain relief with minimal side effects provided the patient is carefully monitored throughout (see below).

PCA devices

There are a variety of battery or electrically operated PCA devices available. Most will include the following features.

- A facility that prevents the device delivering more than the maximum preset dose over a set period, e.g. 4 hours.
- Safety features that include alarms for occlusion (blockage), air in the line, low battery or empty syringe.
- A keypad lock and other locking devices that prevent unauthorised access and changes to the programme.
- An electronic microprocessor that allows the flow rate, bolus dose and lock-out interval to be set. This will usually record the number of bolus doses requested and administered, which is important when determining the effectiveness of the PCA.

An alternative is a mechanical system where a 'control module' is worn around the wrist with a connecting pocket-sized infusor. This is less flexible than the electronic pumps as it only delivers a pre-set, non-adjustable volume and has only one lock-out interval and no safety alarms. However, it is much cheaper than the electronic modes and affords the patient greater freedom of movement.

Patient education

Patient education regarding the use of PCA is vital and with surgical patients, this should occur pre-operatively either in the pre-admission clinic or on the ward. The patient should be encouraged to handle the device and press the buttons, etc., in order to become familiar with the device to be used. It is important that the nurse notes the patient's understanding and dexterity in handling the equipment because patients who are unable to manage the device may not receive any analgesia. If a patient is unable to use the system, nurse-administered analgesia will be required.

Monitoring the patient

Regular monitoring is essential for patients with a PCA. This includes:

1. Close monitoring of respiration rate, particularly immediately after commencement, as respiratory depression is the main side effect of opiate analgesia. Local protocol should be consulted regarding the action to be

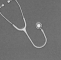

taken if respirations fall below a certain level. A respiratory rate of between 8 and 10 respirations a minute usually requires intervention from the pain control nurse, the anaesthetist or doctor. Some protocols stipulate that patients should have oxygen administered whilst the PCA is in progress. Oxygen saturation levels should be recorded with respiratory rate.

2. The patient's blood pressure, pulse and sedation level should be recorded.
3. Pain should be assessed using a pain assessment tool (see page 33) to ensure effective pain relief is being achieved.
4. The incidence/severity of nausea and vomiting should be recorded.
5. Where possible, patients' usage (i.e. how often they press the button) should be monitored to determine whether the pain control is effective.
6. The prescribed settings for the PCA system should be checked regularly to ensure proper functioning.
7. All of the above should be monitored at least hourly in the early stages. Some areas have a specially designed pain assessment tool that incorporates all of the above areas.
8. The nurse should monitor the infusion site for signs of inflammation, redness or tissue damage (see page 70).
9. As with all controlled drugs, the nurse should prepare, administer and document the infusion in accordance with local trust policy (see page 128).
10. The nurse should ensure no other opiates are administered whilst the patient is receiving PCA.

EPIDURAL ANALGESIA

Principles

Epidural analgesia is an approach to the management of pain in which a fine bore catheter is inserted into the epidural space, the space between the dura mater and the ligaments and bones of the spinal cord. It can be approached at any level of the spine but most commonly at the lumbar or sacral level. The catheter is usually secured to the patient's back using a sterile fixation device and a clear occlusive dressing and is then attached to the infusion device.

The drugs most commonly used for epidural analgesia are opioids (e.g. fentanyl) and local anaesthetics (bupivocaine). Dosages vary according to the site of the catheter, the type of surgery, and the age and medical condition of the patient. Epidural analgesia is commonly used for maternal analgesia during childbirth, and patients who have undergone vascular surgery, thoracic or abdominal surgery, or orthopaedic surgery to the lower limb.

Monitoring patients with epidural analgesia

Careful monitoring of the patient is vital and includes the following.

- The prescribed settings on the epidural device or pump must be checked regularly to ensure it is functioning properly. The device should never be regarded as fail-safe.

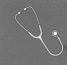

- Single luer-lock connections must be used between the catheter and the administration set. Three-way connectors must not be used to prevent inadvertent administration of other medications.
- A bacterial filter must be in place at the end of the epidural cannula.
- The epidural cannula must be clearly labelled.
- Close monitoring of sedation levels. Sedation and respiratory depression are known side effects of opioids. The use of a sedation score is recommended to assist in the early detection of respiratory depression. If the score signifies the patient is becoming unacceptably sedated, the infusion should be stopped and oxygen administered whilst medical or anaesthetic intervention is sought.
- Close monitoring of respirations should be undertaken alongside sedation scores. Oxygen saturation levels are recorded with respiratory rate, although they should not be used as the primary or only indicator of respiratory depression.
- Patients receiving opioids can develop pruritus (itching) that is distressing and does not always respond to antihistamines. If the itching does not respond to intervention, the opioid may need to be discontinued.
- The blood pressure and pulse rate should be recorded hourly. Hypotension is associated with the use of local anaesthetics in epidural analgesia and can also occur if the epidural catheter migrates into the subarachnoid space. This would be accompanied by light-headedness, tachycardia (raised pulse) and difficulty with movement. The infusion should be stopped and medical assistance sought immediately if any of these symptoms occur.
- Local anaesthetics can also be toxic to the central nervous systems. The nurse should assess the patient excitation, numbness of the tongue and mouth, slurred speech, twitching, light-headedness and tinnitus (buzzing or ringing in the ears). If central nervous system toxicity occurs the patient may experience respiratory depression, convulsions and is at risk of cardiac arrest. If toxicity is suspected the infusion must be stopped. The priority of medical intervention is the patient's ventilation and oxygen needs.
- Fluid intake should be monitored to ensure that any reduction in blood pressure is not associated with dehydration. Where possible, oral fluids must be encouraged and intravenous infusion considered.
- Urinary output must be monitored, particularly in those patients with lumbar epidural analgesia as it is commonly associated with urinary retention. If the patient has a urinary catheter, hourly measurements should be undertaken. Accurate recording on a fluid balance chart is essential.
- The height of the epidural block can be assessed by the application of cold to the skin surface. If the patient reports pins and needles in the fingers this should be reported. The hourly rate of the infusion may need to be reduced.
- Pain should be assessed using a pain assessment tool to ensure effective pain relief is being achieved. If the patient reports pain at the site of the infusion, medical staff should be informed as infection or haematoma may be present.
- Nausea and vomiting (often using a scoring system) should be recorded.
- All of the above should be monitored simultaneously and hourly for the duration of the epidural analgesia. Some areas have a specially designed assessment tool.

- As with all controlled drugs, the nurse must prepare, administer and document the drugs according to the local policy (see page 128). No other opiates should be prescribed or administered while epidural analgesia is in progress.

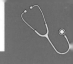

Bibliography/Suggested reading

Temperature, pulse and blood pressure recording

Blows W T. *The biological basis of nursing: clinical observations.* London: Routledge; 2001.

Connell F. The causes and treatment of fever: a literature review. *Nursing Standard* 1997, **12**(11):40–43.

Edwards S. Measuring temperature. *Professional Nurse Study Supplement* 1997, **3**(2):5–7.

Edwards S. Recording blood pressure. *Professional Nurse Study Supplement* 1997, **13**(2):8–10.

Erickson R, Meyer L. Accuracy of infrared tympanic and other temperature methods in adults. *American Journal of Critical Care* 1994, **3**(1):40–54.

Fulbrook P. Core temperature measurement in adults: a literature review. *Journal of Advanced Nursing* 1993; **18**(9):1451–1460.

Jevon P. Using a tympanic thermometer. *Nursing Times* 2001, **97**(9):43–44

O'Brien E, Davison M. Blood pressure measurement: rational and ritual actions. *British Journal of Nursing* 1994, **3**(8):393–396.

O'Brien E, Petrie J, Littler W. *Blood pressure measurement: recommendations of the British Hypertension Society.* London: British Medical Journal Publishing Group; 1997.

O'Toole S. Alternatives to mercury thermometers. *Professional Nurse* 1997, **12**(11):783–786.

Skinner S. *Understanding clinical investigations.* London: Baillière Tindall; 1996.

Toms E. Vital observations. *Nursing Times* 1995, **89**(51):32–34.

Woollons S. Temperature measurement devices. *Professional Nurse* 1996, **11**(8):541–542, 544–547.

Care of seizures

Brodie MJ. Status epilepticus in adults. *Lancet* 1990, **336**:551–555.

Board M. Comparison of disposable and glass mercury thermometers. *Nursing Times* 1995, **91**(33):36–37.

Sung C, Chu N. Epileptic seizures in elderly people: aetiology and seizure type. *Age and Ageing* 1990, **19**(1):25–30.

Cardiac monitoring and ECG

Docherty B, Roe J. Cardiac arrhythmias: recognition and care. *Professional Nurse* 2001, **16**:1492–1496.

Jevon P, Ewens B (eds). *Monitoring the critically ill patient.* Oxford: Blackwell Science Ltd; 2002.

Pope B. How to perform 3-or-5-lead monitoring. *Nursing* 2002, **32**(4):5550–5552

Assessment of level of consciousness

Blows W T. *The biological basis of nursing: clinical observations.* London: Routledge; 2001.

Shah S. Neurological assessment (RCN Continuing Education). *Nursing Standard* 1999, **13**(22):49–56.

Stewart N. Neurological observations. *Professional Nurse* 1996, **11**(6): 377–378.

Weighing patients

Harrison M. Weighty concerns (research on accuracy of weighing procedures and equipment in hospitals). *Nursing Times* 1991, **87**(42):40–42.

Blood glucose monitoring

Burden M. Diabetes: blood glucose monitoring. *Nursing Times* 2001, **97**(8):36–39.

Lowes L. Accuracy in ward-based blood glucose monitoring. *Nursing Times* 1995, **91**(13):44–45.

Neurovascular observation

Eden-Kilgour S, Miller B. Understanding neurovascular assessment. *Nursing* 1993, **23**(8):56–58.

Pain assessment

Broadbent C. The pharmacology of acute pain. *Nursing Times* 2000, **96**(26):39–41.

Cowan T. Patient-controlled analgesia devices. *Professional Nurse* 1997, **13**(2):119–123.

Cox F. Clinical care of patients with epidural infusion. *Professional Nurse* 2001, **16**:1429–1432.

Cox F. Making sense of epidural analgesia. *Nursing Times* 2002, **98**(32): NT Plus Pain supplement, pp 56–58.

Craig KD. Emotional aspects of pain. In: Wall PD, Melzack R (eds). *Textbook of pain.* Edinburgh: Churchill Livingstone; 1989.

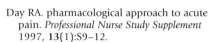
Day RA. pharmacological approach to acute pain. *Professional Nurse Study Supplement* 1997, **13**(1):S9–12.

Hall GM, Salmon P. Patient-controlled analgesia: who benefits? (Editorial) *Anaesthesia* 1997, **52**:401.

Lawler K. Pain assessment. *Professional Nurse Study Supplement* 1997, **13**(1):S5–8.

Lynch M. Pain as the fifth vital sign. *Journal of Intravenous Nursing* 2001, **24**(2):85–94.

Macintyre PE, Ready LB. *Acute pain management: a practical guide.* London: WB Saunders Co; 1996.

Thomas N. Patient-controlled analgesia. *Nursing Standard* 1996, **10**(47):49–55.

2

Resuscitation

Preparation

Patient

- The patient is unresponsive when called or shaken.

Equipment/Environment

- No equipment is necessary.

Nurse

- Behave calmly.

Procedure

1. **Approach** the patient/surroundings carefully to exclude any risk of danger to yourself, e.g. electrical cable. There may be something to indicate the possible cause of collapse (e.g. fall or injury).
2. **Assess** the patient's conscious state. Shake the patient (unless possible neck injury) and shout (in both ears) to see if they respond.
3. If the person is unconscious (i.e. totally unresponsive) call for help from a bystander (if present) and ask them to wait while you complete your assessment.
4. **Airway** – with one hand tip back the forehead and with the other, open the mouth to observe whether there is any obvious obstruction. Remove any visible obstruction but leave well-fitting dentures in place. Using two fingers under the point of the chin, lift the chin to raise the tongue from the back of the throat to clear the airway (see Figure 2.3). Keep it raised.
5. **Breathing** – place your cheek near the patient's nostrils to **feel** for any breathing. **Look** for chest movement and **listen** for breath sounds. Observe for about 10 seconds. If no breathing is detected, start basic life support (see page 44). If breathing is present, place the casualty in the recovery position (see below).

Recovery position

1. Place the person in the recovery position – i.e. on their side, with the lower arm at 90° to the body and the back of uppermost hand under the cheek. The uppermost knee should be bent to prevent the person rolling onto their stomach (Figure 2.1).
2. Send for help unless recovery is immediate **PFP1** .
3. Continue to observe the person carefully, to ensure that breathing and circulation are being maintained.

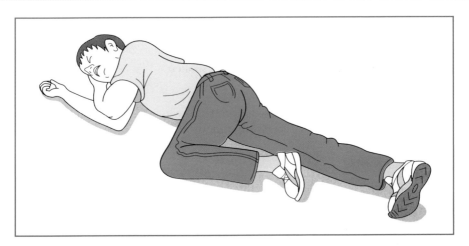

Figure 2.1 Recovery position

Points for practice

1. If the collapse has occurred in the street or someone's home, send for an ambulance. If it is in a hospital or nursing home, refer to local policy.

Preparation

Patient

• The patient is unresponsive when called or shaken.

Equipment/Environment

• Some people carry a pocket resuscitation mask, which may be used to prevent contact with the person's saliva during mouth-to-mouth respiration in an emergency (Figure 2.2).

Nurse

• Yearly updating in resuscitation techniques is vital to maintain these skills.

Procedure

1. **Approach** the patient/surroundings carefully to exclude any risk of danger to yourself, e.g. electrical cable. There may be something to indicate the possible cause of collapse (e.g. fall or injury).
2. **Assess** the patient's conscious state. Shake the patient (unless possible neck injury) and shout in both ears to see if they respond.
3. If the person is unconscious (i.e. totally unresponsive) call for help from a bystander (if present) and ask them to wait while you complete your assessment.
4. **Airway** – with one hand tip back the forehead and with the other, open the mouth to observe whether there is any obvious obstruction. Remove any visible obstruction but leave well-fitting dentures in place. Using two fingers under the point of the chin, lift the chin to raise the tongue from the back of the throat to clear the airway (see Figure 2.3). Keep it raised.

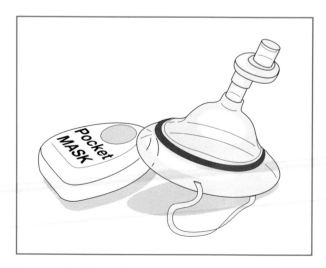

Figure 2.2 Pocket resuscitation mask

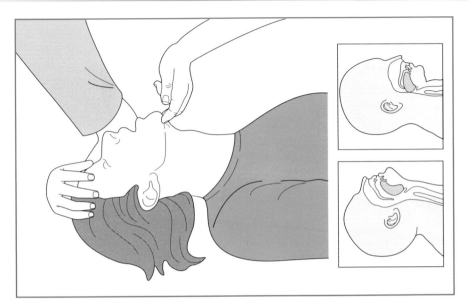

Figure 2.3 Chin lifted to bring tongue forward from back of throat

5. **Breathing** – place your cheek near the patient's nostrils to **feel** for any breathing. **Look** for chest movement and **listen** for breath sounds. Observe for about 10 seconds.
6. If the person is breathing, place them in the recovery position (see page 42). If the person is not breathing, send for help (or go yourself if no-one else is around) and then commence cardiopulmonary resuscitation (CPR, see below) **PFP1** .

Cardiopulmonary resuscitation

1. Make sure the mouth and airway is clear (keep well-fitting dentures in).
2. Commence mouth-to-mouth breathing – keeping the chin lifted, pinch the patient's nose and place your lips around the patient's open mouth. Give two steady rescue breaths, watching each time to see the chest rising **PFP2,3** .
3. Feel for a carotid pulse for up to 10 seconds. If no pulse is felt, commence external cardiac compressions **PFP4,5,6** .
   • Identify the tip of the sternum. With your middle finger on the point where the ribs join the sternum, place your index finger on the sternum (Figure 2.4A) and place the heel of your other hand on the sternum next to your index finger (in men the position is in a line between the nipples).
   • Remove your index finger, and place this hand on top of the other and interlock the fingers, keeping them raised off the chest wall (see Figure 2.4B).
   • With the arms straight, press down 4–5 cm and release, firmly and rhythmically, counting aloud 1, 2, 3, etc., to 15 compressions (Figure 2.4C).
4. Repeat two effective breaths and continue at a ratio of two breaths to 15 compressions until help arrives.

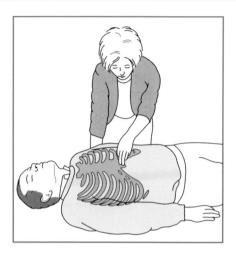
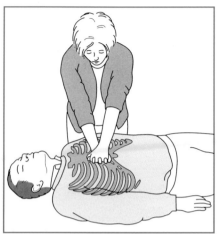
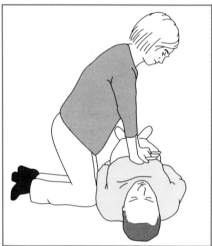

Figure 2.4 Cardiac compressions
A = Identifying the tip of the sternum
B = Hands in position for cardiac compressions
C = Cardiac compressions

Post procedure

Patient

• Once help arrives, the experienced professionals will take over from you.

Nurse

• Cardiopulmonary resuscitation is physically and emotionally exhausting. Try to talk through what happened with someone afterwards.
• Despite your best efforts, the person may not survive.

Points for practice

1. If there is no-one to send for help, go yourself. Then return and start cardiopulmonary resuscitation.

2. The chest should rise with every breath. If it does not, check the mouth again for visible obstruction and make sure the chin is still lifted to bring the tongue forward. If after five attempts two effective breaths have still not been achieved (i.e. the chest is seen to rise), proceed to assess the circulation.

3. Do not over-breathe as this may inflate the stomach and cause vomiting. Wait for the chest to fall after each breath before giving another breath.

4. Look for signs of circulation. Feel for the carotid pulse if you have been trained to do so. The carotid pulse is nearest to the heart. If no pulse can be felt here, there is no cardiac output.

5. In the case of respiratory arrest causing the heart to stop (as in drowning), the heart may restart, so feel for the pulse during resuscitation if the colour changes greatly.

6. Resuscitation techniques are reviewed regularly. It is important to ensure that you have knowledge of the most up-to-date guidelines.

Preparation

Patient

Check:

- Unconscious.
- Not breathing.
- No pulse.
- Is the patient for resuscitation PFP1 .

Equipment/Environment

- Emergency equipment box or trolley including emergency drugs box.
- Gloves, goggles and plastic aprons (usually kept with emergency equipment).
- Oxygen cylinder (if piped oxygen is not available).
- Suction machine (if piped suction is not available).
- Intravenous (IV) infusion stand.
- ECG monitor and defibrillator.
- Screen bed area to maintain privacy.

Nurse

- Summon help PFP2 .
- The most experienced nurse should co-ordinate the activities of other staff.
- If sufficient staff are available, delegate someone to care for the other patients.

Procedure

1. Lay the patient flat. If in bed, remove pillows and the head of the bed PFP3 .
2. Lift the chin to open the airway and check there is no obstruction. Give two effective rescue breaths (i.e. effective inflations). If there is no carotid pulse, commence cardiopulmonary resuscitation at a ratio of two breaths to 15 compressions.
3. Once available, insert an appropriate sized oropharyngeal (Guedel) airway PFP4 . Insert it into the mouth upside down and then turn it into position over the back of the tongue (Figure 2.5). Attach oxygen tubing to the Ambu bag and set oxygen flow to 10L per minute PFP5 .
4. Holding the chin up and the face mask tight against the face (Figure 2.6), compress the Ambu bag at a steady speed. Check that the chest is rising with each 'breath', i.e. compression of the bag. Give two 'breaths' after every 15 cardiac compressions.
5. Continue 15 external cardiac compressions after every two 'breaths'.
6. When the medical/senior nursing team arrive, the following may be instigated according to the condition of the patient:
   - Endotracheal intubation – check the suction machine is working and has an oral sucker attached. Once the patient is intubated, a tracheal suction catheter will be required.
   - IV cannulation (often internal/external jugular) to enable drugs such as adrenaline (epinephrine) to be given intravenously.

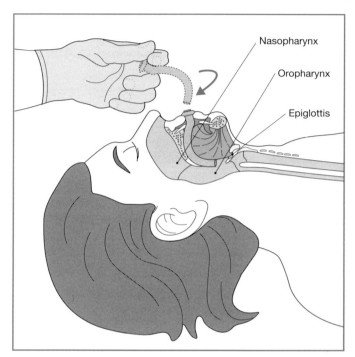

Nasopharynx

Oropharynx

Epiglottis

Figure 2.5 Position of oropharyngeal (Guedel) airway

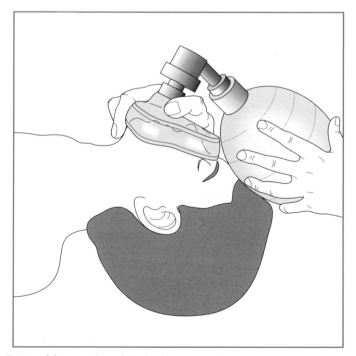

Figure 2.6 Use of face mask and Ambu bag

- ECG monitoring/recording.
- Defibrillation.
7. The timing of each event and the administration of any drugs must be recorded.

Post procedure

Patient

- If resuscitation is successful, close monitoring of the patient's condition will be necessary and the patient may be transferred to an intensive care unit.
- If resuscitation is unsuccessful, ensure privacy and dignity are maintained and prepare the patient to be seen by the family.

Equipment/Environment

- Emergency equipment must be cleaned and restocked immediately and made ready for use.
- Dispose of used equipment according to local policy.

Nurse

- Document the event in the nursing records.
- All involved should discuss the way the situation was managed **PFP6** .

Points for practice

1. Resuscitation is not appropriate in some patients. The situation must be discussed with the patient and/or the family and if a decision has been made not to resuscitate, this must be written in the medical notes by the patient's medical consultant. It should also be written in the nursing documentation and communicated at every shift handover.

2. In a hospital, there will be a Resuscitation Team, who can be summoned urgently by phoning a special number. It is vital to check that you know the emergency number in every area that you work. The ward may also have an emergency buzzer system to summon help.

3. If the patient is on a pressure-relieving mattress, there is a quick-release mechanism to enable rapid deflation in an emergency.

4. The Guedel airway is designed to hold the tongue forward to prevent it obstructing the airway. The correct size is determined by choosing an airway that is the same length as the distance from the tip of the patient's ear to the corner of his/her mouth.

5. Oxygen may be given without prescription in an emergency situation.

6. If the resuscitation is unsuccessful, it can be distressing for all involved and time should be allowed to support junior staff and talk it through.

Bibliography/Suggested reading

Pertab D. Basic life support techniques in adults. *Professional Nurse* 1999, **15**(1):37–41.

Playfer J. 'Not for resuscitation' – whose decision? *Geriatric Medicine* 1994, **24**(5):21.

Resuscitation Council UK. *Resuscitation guidelines*. London: Resuscitation Council UK; 2000.

Winser H. An evidence base for adult resuscitation. *Professional Nurse* 2001, **16**:1120–1213.

Notes

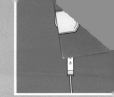

3

IV therapy

Preparation

Patient

- Explain the procedure, to gain consent and co-operation.
- The patient should be sitting or lying comfortably, with the appropriate arm supported. Clothing may need to be removed to allow access to the arm.

Equipment/Environment

- Green needle (21G) and syringe (size will vary according to the amount of blood needed) and blood sample tubes as appropriate, or vacuum tube sampling system and appropriate sample tubes.
- Skin-cleansing agent.
- Tourniquet.
- Gauze swabs or cotton-wool balls.
- Small self-adhesive dressing.
- Sharps bin.

Nurse

- Hands must be washed and dried thoroughly.
- Gloves (close-fitting to allow dexterity) should be worn.

Procedure

1. Check the patient's identity with the blood test request form and ask/assist patient to adjust clothing as necessary.
2. Assemble all equipment. Do not label the sample tubes until the blood specimen is in them **PFP1** .
3. Inspect the arm to select a suitable vein **PFP2** and apply the tourniquet **PFP3** . Palpate the vein to locate its position and ensure that it is not an artery (which will pulsate) or a tendon.
4. Clean the skin with the skin-cleansing agent and allow to dry completely **PFP4** .
5. With the patient's arm straight and well supported, use your non-dominant hand to pull the skin tight over the vein to 'anchor' the vein.
6. Take the syringe and needle (or needle and plastic holder of vacuum-type system) in your dominant hand. With the bevel of the needle upward and directly over the vein, insert the needle at an angle of about 15° through the skin and into the vein.
7. **Needle and syringe** – blood will appear at the tip of the syringe to indicate that the vein has been punctured. Hold the needle in position with one hand and with the other steadily pull back the piston of the syringe until the required amount of blood is obtained (Figure 3.1A). Do not pull too vigorously or the vein may collapse.

Vacuum system – after puncturing the vein, no blood is visible until the sample tube is attached. Hold the needle and plastic holder securely in place and attach the sample tube by pushing it firmly onto the needle attachment inside the holder (Figure 3.1B). The tube will then automatically fill with blood to the required amount. If additional samples are required, remove the tube when full (no blood will leak out) and attach another.

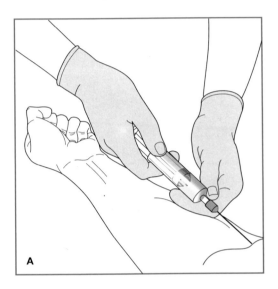

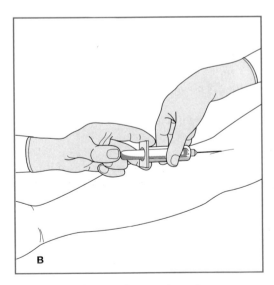

Figure 3.1 A = Venepuncture using a syringe and needle
B = Venepuncture using a vacuum system

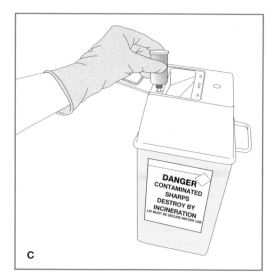

C

Figure 3.1 C = Using the non-touch needle-removing device

8. Remove the tourniquet, hold the gauze swab or cotton-wool ball over the puncture site and remove the needle. Do not press until the needle is out of the vein as this is very painful for the patient. Continue to apply pressure (or ask the patient to do this) for 2–3 minutes until the bleeding stops, to prevent bruising.
9. **Needle and syringe** – using the non-touch needle-removing device on the sharps bin (Figure 3.1C), remove the needle from the syringe before transferring the blood to the sample tube **PFP5** .

    Vacuum system – using the non-touch needle-removing device on the sharps bin (Figure 3.1C). Remove the needle and discard. If appropriate, retain the plastic holder for future use **PFP6** .

Post procedure

Patient

- Ask the patient to continue pressing but not to bend the arm as this may cause a haematoma. Once the bleeding has stopped, apply a small self-adhesive dressing.
- Assist the patient to replace clothing as necessary.

Equipment/Environment

- Discard all sharps and other waste safely.

Nurse

- Remove gloves and wash hands.
- Label specimens with the patient's surname, first names, hospital number, date of birth, ward/clinic and the date of the sample.

Points for practice

1. Do not label the sample tubes in advance in case venepuncture is unsuccessful and the tubes are mistakenly used for another patient.

2. The best veins are usually found at the elbow, in the antecubital fossa. These veins are less mobile, easier to puncture and less painful than veins in the hand or lower arm. If the patient is very cold, it may help to ask the patient to warm their hands in warm water for a few minutes or clench and unclench a fist several times to increase blood flow to the arm. Gently tapping the vein may also increase vasodilation by causing histamine release at the site. This must be gentle as vigorous tapping may cause venous spasm.

3. The tourniquet should not be applied for longer than 1 minute before collecting the blood specimen. Prolonged use will cause intravascular fluid to leak into the tissues and may affect the accuracy of the blood test.

4. The skin-cleansing agent is usually alcohol-based and must be allowed to dry completely before proceeding. Any residual alcohol causes pain for the patient and may damage the cells and affect the blood specimen.

5. Cells may be damaged if the blood is squirted through the needle into the sample tube. Damage can cause them to leak potassium and may lead to an inaccurate result.

6. Refer to local policy regarding re-use of the plastic holder. It should always be discussed if it becomes contaminated with blood or the patient has an infection such as hepatitis or MRSA.

Preparation

Patient

- Explain the procedure, to gain consent and co-operation.
- The patient should be sitting or lying comfortably, with the appropriate arm (non-dominant if possible) supported. If the cannula is for an IV infusion or the clothing is tight or restrictive, remove the arm from the sleeve.
- Local anaesthetic cream, if used, must be applied at least 1 hour prior to the procedure PFP1 .
- Cannulation will be easier if the patient's arms and hands are warm and well perfused.

Equipment/Environment

- Tourniquet.
- Skin-cleansing agent (e.g. chlorhexidine in alcohol) according to local policy.
- Cannula of appropriate size PFP2 – check the expiry date and that the packaging is intact.
- Sterile cannula dressing.
- Ten millilitres of 0.9% sodium chloride to flush the cannula (check the expiry date).
- Injectable cap or prepared infusion ready to connect (see page 61).
- Disposable pad or towel to place under the arm to protect the bed linen.
- Sharps bin.
- Environment should ensure warmth, privacy and adequate lighting.

Nurse

- Hands must be washed and dried thoroughly.
- Gloves (close-fitting to allow dexterity) and an apron should be worn.

Procedure

1. If possible, choose the patient's non-dominant arm for cannulation. Place towel or pad under the arm.
2. Apply the tourniquet 5–10 cm above the proposed site of cannulation and check for arterial blood flow. If the tourniquet is so tight that it prevents arterial blood flow, the veins will not fill.
3. Ask the patient to clench and unclench their fist several times to encourage venous filling. Gently tapping the vein may also encourage vasodilation by causing histamine release at the site. Select a vein by palpation, not just visually, to ensure that it is suitable (i.e. bouncy not hard) and is not an artery (which will pulsate) or a tendon PFP3 .
4. Clean the site with cleansing agent and allow to dry. Do not touch the site again with your fingers.
5. Take the cannula and check that the needle can be removed easily, but do not remove it. Hold the cannula in your dominant hand with the sharp bevelled end facing upwards (Figure 3.2).

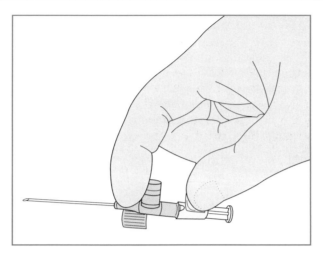

Figure 3.2 Cannula with bevel upwards

6. With your other hand, hold the patient's arm and 'anchor' the vein with your thumb, just below the selected insertion site, to prevent it moving when punctured.
7. Holding the cannula at an angle of 20–30° either directly over the vein or just to one side of it, insert the cannula through the skin and into the vein **PFP4**.
8. Stop advancing the cannula as soon as it is in the vein (blood will appear at the end of the cannula when it enters the vein) and lower the angle of the cannula.
9. Holding the needle part of the cannula with one hand to stop it advancing any further (and going right through the vein), slide the cannula off the needle and into the vein with the other hand.
10. Hold the cannula in place to prevent dislodgement and release the tourniquet. Place a piece of sterile gauze under the end of the cannula to contain any drops of blood during removal of the needle (step 13).
11. If an injectable cap is being used, open the packaging (taking care not to contaminate the sterile end) and hold it between the thumb and forefinger of your dominant hand. If an infusion is to be connected, see page 61.
12. With your other hand, apply pressure to the vein immediately above the end of the cannula to minimise blood flow (Figure 3.3).
13. Remove the needle and swiftly insert the injectable cap or the administration set of the infusion.
14. Clean up any blood and apply the sterile dressing **PFP5**, ensuring that the cannula is held securely in place.
15. Flush the cannula with 0.9% sodium chloride to ensure patency.

Post procedure

Patient

- Explain any restrictions to mobility and the need to protect the cannula site.
- Instruct the patient to report any swelling, redness or pain.

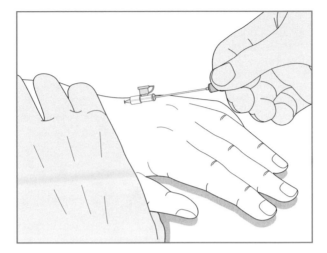

Figure 3.3 Hand applying pressure before withdrawing the needle

Equipment/Environment

- Discard sharps and other clinical waste safely.
- Return sharps bin and tourniquet to the appropriate places.

Nurse

- Remove gloves and apron and wash hands.
- Document cannulation in the nursing records.

Points for practice

1. Although most adult patients will not require it, local anaesthetic may be desirable with patients who are extremely anxious or needle-phobic. Local anaesthetic cream must be applied at least 1 hour in advance to be effective. The use of injected local anaesthetic is debatable as this requires a needle-prick and may make the selected vein more difficult to see.

2. The size of cannula required will be determined by the type of fluid to be infused and the size and condition of the patient's veins. The smallest gauge capable of achieving the required flow rate should be used.

3. If it is difficult to palpate the vein with gloves on, do this without gloves and then put them on once the vein is identified.

4. Despite 'anchoring' with the thumb, the vein sometimes moves when directly punctured from above. Consequently, many people prefer to insert the cannula through the skin slightly to one side of the vein and then direct it into the vein.

5. The type of dressing used will be dictated by local policy. Non-sterile tape should not be used to secure the cannula as this has been shown to increase the risk of infection.

Preparation

Patient

• Explain the reasons for IV infusion and any limitations to mobility.

Equipment/Environment

• IV infusion fluid according to the prescription.
• IV administration set of appropriate type **PFP1**.
• IV infusion stand.

Nurse

• Wash and dry hands throughly.

Procedure

Intravenous fluid

1. The IV fluid to be administered must be checked by a registered nurse **PFP2,3**. Blood transfusions require special checking procedure (see page 88).
2. Check the outer wrapper is intact and not damaged in any way.
3. Open the outer wrapper and remove the bag.
4. Check the fluid bag for leakage, particles, cloudiness, expiry date and batch number.

Administration set

1. Check the contents are sterile, i.e. the outer wrapper is not damaged or wet.
2. Check the expiry date/date of sterilisation.
3. Open the packaging and remove the administration set. Both ends should be covered with protective caps to maintain sterility.
4. Close the flow control clamp on the administration set.

Assembly

1. Remove the protective cap from the insertion port on the bag of fluid and hold carefully to maintain sterility.
2. Remove the protective cover from the spike of the administration set (just above the drip chamber).
3. Taking care to maintain sterility, insert the spike into the bag, pushing and twisting until fully inserted (see Figure 3.5).
4. Hang the bag on the infusion stand. Squeeze and release the drip chamber until it is half-full of fluid.
5. Partially open the roller clamp to allow fluid to run through the set, thus expelling the air (not too quickly or it will draw in air from the drip chamber).
6. When all the air has been expelled, close the roller clamp. The infusion is now ready for use.
7. Taking care to maintain sterility, remove the protective cap from the administration set and the cap from the cannula. Swiftly connect the set and 'lock' into position.

8. Secure tubing with tape to prevent pulling (see Figure 3.7 on page 71) and adjust the roller clamp to set the infusion to the prescribed rate (see page 66).

Post procedure

Patient

- Ensure the patient is comfortable and understands about the infusion.
- Instruct the patient to report any swelling, redness or pain.

Equipment/Environment

- Discard all packaging into the clinical waste system.

Nurse

- Record the time the infusion started and the batch number of the IV fluid according to local policy.
- Document the care in the nursing records.

Points for practice

1. The type of administration set used will depend upon the type of fluid being administered. Blood and blood products require an administration set with a filter (Figure 3.4B) that incorporates a 170µm filter to remove microaggregates that are formed during storage of the blood (Bradbury & Cruickshank 2000). Clear fluids require a simple administration set without a filter chamber (Figure 3.4A).

2. In most cases, all IV fluids must be checked by a registered nurse, although this may vary according to local policy. In some Trusts, two nurses are required to check IV fluid. Procedures for checking blood transfusions are detailed on page 88.

3. Infusions requiring great accuracy will be controlled through an IV pump or syringe driver. A burette (Figure 3.4C) may be used to administer small amounts of fluid or drugs. They are always used with children to prevent accidental over-infusion.

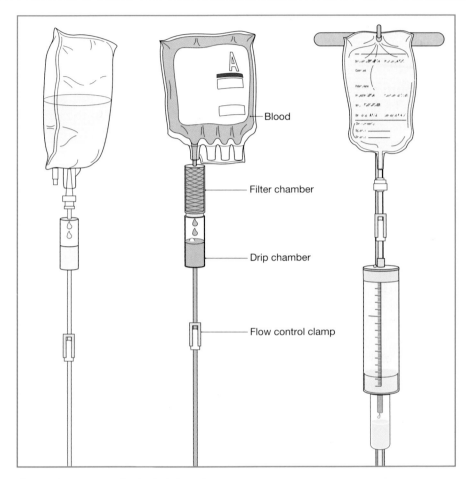

Blood

Filter chamber

Drip chamber

Flow control clamp

Figure 3.4 A = Standard administration set
B = Blood administration set
C = Burette

Changing an infusion bag

Preparation

Patient

- Explain the procedure.

Equipment/Environment

- IV infusion fluid as prescribed.
- For blood transfusions see page 91.

Nurse

- The hands must be washed and dried thoroughly.
- The infusion fluid must be checked by a registered nurse.

Procedure

1. Remove the infusion fluid from its outer wrapper and check the fluid bag for leakage, particles, cloudiness, expiry date, volume and batch number.
2. Ensure that it is the correct infusion fluid by checking it with the prescription chart and the patient's identity. (NB This must be checked by a registered nurse, see page 88.)
3. Close the roller clamp on the administration set.
4. Remove the empty infusion bag from the stand and pull out the spike of the administration set, taking care not to contaminate it.
5. Remove the protective cover from the inlet port of the new infusion bag and insert the spike of the giving set, twisting until fully inserted (Figure 3.5).
6. Replace the bag on the infusion stand and adjust the roller clamp to the prescribed flow rate (see page 66).

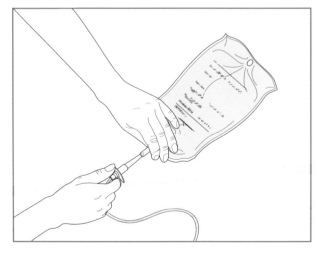

Figure 3.5 Inserting the spike of the administration set into the new infusion bag

Post procedure

Patient

- Check at least hourly that the infusion is running as prescribed and the patient is not complaining of pain or discomfort at the site.
- Observe the patient for signs of fluid overload (rising pulse and respiratory rate).

Equipment/Environment

- Discard the used infusion bag and packaging into the clinical waste system.

Nurse

- Document the infusion (amount, type of fluid, time commenced, batch number and signature of the nurse) according to local policy.
- If the patient has a fluid chart, the infusion should be recorded on this according to local policy **PFP1**.

Points for practice

1. Most patients with an IV infusion will require a fluid balance chart to monitor fluid input and output (see page 169). The new infusion and completion of the old infusion should be recorded.

Principles

The use of IV devices (pumps and syringe drivers) to regulate infusions is steadily increasing in general-ward areas. However, a large number of simple infusions will be regulated using gravity and the roller clamp only (Figure 3.6). It is important that infusions run at a constant rate over the prescribed time.

Calculating the flow rate in 'drops per minute'

If it is a simple gravity infusion, or an infusion device that regulates the flow rate in 'drops per minute' is being used, calculation of the rate in drops per minute is necessary **PFP1**. The calculation is as follows:

$$\frac{\text{volume of infusion in ml} \times \text{number of drops per ml}}{\text{time in minutes}} = \text{flow rate in drops per minute}$$

The number of drops per ml will be determined by the administration set being used and is indicated on the packaging:

- Standard administration set = 20 drops per ml.
- Blood administration set = 15 drops per ml.
- Paediatric set (burette) = 60 drops per ml.

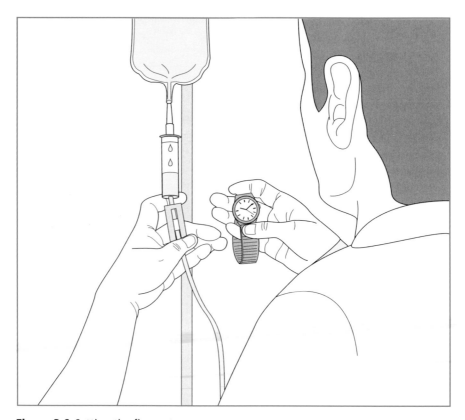

Figure 3.6 Setting the flow rate

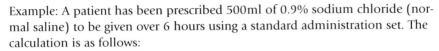

Example: A patient has been prescribed 500ml of 0.9% sodium chloride (normal saline) to be given over 6 hours using a standard administration set. The calculation is as follows:

$$\frac{\textbf{500}\ (\text{vol of infusion}) \times \textbf{20}\ (\text{N}^\circ \text{ of drops per ml})}{\textbf{360}\ (6\ \text{hours} \times 60\ \text{minutes})} = \frac{500 \times 20}{360} = \frac{10\ 000}{360}$$

$$= 27.77\ \text{drops per minute (round up to 28)}$$

Example: A patient has been prescribed 420ml of whole blood to be given over 4 hours using a blood administration set. The calculation is as follows:

$$\frac{420 \times 15}{240} = \frac{6300}{240} = 26.25\ \text{drops per minte (round up to 27 drops)}$$

Calculating the flow rate in 'millilitres per hour'

If a volumetric infusion pump or syringe driver is being used, it is necessary to calculate the number of millilitres required per hour. The calculation is as follows:

$$\frac{\text{volume of infusion in ml}}{\text{no. of hours}} = \text{flow rate in millititres per hour}$$

Example: A patient has been prescribed 1 litre of 5% dextrose to be given over 8 hours. The calculation is as follows:

$$\frac{1000}{8} = 125\text{ml per hour}$$

Points for practice

1. You are likely to be using a calculator for these calculations. It is important that you check your answer several times to ensure that you have used the correct maths. If you are working with junior nurses, it is important to be able to demonstrate your calculation, to enable them to learn.

Principles

IV pumps and syringe drivers are increasingly being used to control infusions in general wards as well as in specialist areas. There are a large number of different types available from a range of manufacturers and a detailed description of each will be found in the manufacturer's users' manual. To guarantee safe and accurate practice, nurses have a responsibility to ensure that they are familiar with any equipment being used. If unsure of any aspect of the pump or syringe driver, it is important to seek help from a more experienced nurse or from the hospital department where IV devices are maintained. Although IV devices may differ in appearance, there are a number of features that are likely to be common to all. Make sure you are familiar with the following features on the syringe driver or pump you are using.

Power supply

- Is the device powered by battery, mains electricity or both?
- If batteries, what type are they?
- If it has a rechargeable battery: how long will it run on the battery?; how is the battery charged?; how do you know when it needs charging?

Administration set/cassette/syringe

- Most devices can only be used with a specific administration set, cassette or type of syringe.
- If it is possible to use different sizes and types, how does the device confirm recognition of the type being used?

Setting up the device

- You must be familiar with the correct procedure for setting up the device. All administration sets, cassettes and syringes are designed to be inserted easily into the device. If force is required, the correct procedure is not being followed.

Alarm systems

- Most devices have a number of alarms to alert the nurse to situations such as 'air in the line', 'infusion complete' and 'occlusion of the line'.
- Most will have a mute button to allow the alarm to be silenced while dealing with the problem. It is vital that alarms are never turned off (however irritating), as dangerous situations may then go undetected.
- If any alarm feature is not working properly, the device must not be used.
- Some smaller devices do not have any alarms and so they must be checked at least once every hour to ensure safe and accurate administration of the drug or infusion.

Maintenance and repair

- All IV devices must be maintained regularly to ensure safe and accurate use. Most hospitals have a system of regular maintenance indicated by a sticker on the device, showing the date when maintenance is due. Pumps and syringe drivers must not be used after this date and should be returned to the relevant department for maintenance.

- Most devices that are powered by mains electricity also have a battery for short-term use when transferring a patient or during a power cut. The device should be kept plugged into the mains at all times, even when not in use, to ensure the battery remains fully charged.

Preparation

Patient

- Inspect the cannula site to determine whether the dressing needs changing PFP1 .
- Explain the procedure, to gain consent and co-operation.
- The patient must be able to co-operate by keeping the arm very still during the dressing, to prevent accidental dislodgement. If there is doubt, assistance may be required.

Equipment/Environment

- The cannula site should be considered as a wound and so should not be exposed unnecessarily or during bed making, dusting, etc.
- Sterile dressing – the type will vary according to local policy but it should be one that is specially designed for IV cannulae.
- If the cannula site requires cleaning, a small dressing pack will be required plus cleansing solution according to local policy.

Nurse

- The hands must be washed and dried thoroughly.
- As there is a risk of direct contact with blood, gloves should be worn. These should be close-fitting gloves to enable manipulation of self-adhesive dressing and tape.
- A plastic apron should also be worn.

Procedure

1. Ensure that all equipment is within easy reach. Protect the area under the arm with a disposable dressing towel or similar, to collect any spillage.
2. Explain to the patient the importance of remaining still during the procedure, to prevent dislodgement of the cannula.
3. Maintaining asepsis, open the pack and new dressing and pour the cleansing solution (see aseptic dressing technique, page 222).
4. Put on the sterile gloves and using the sterile disposal bag as a 'glove' (see page 223), carefully remove the old dressing, taking care not to dislodge the cannula. Assistance may be required to secure the cannula during this procedure.
5. If necessary, clean the cannula site PFP2 . Inspect the site for signs of phlebitis, infection, and other problems (redness, swelling, etc).
6. Apply the new dressing, taking care not to touch the part that will be directly over the insertion site PFP3 .
7. If an IV infusion is running, secure the tubing of the administration set to prevent pulling and accidental dislodgement of the cannula (Figure 3.7).

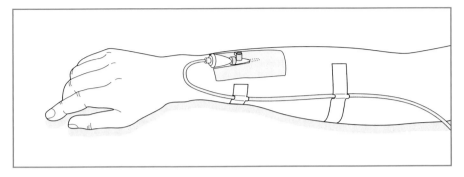

Figure 3.7 Securing the intravenous tubing

Post procedure

Patient

• Ensure comfort and check understanding regarding the IV site.

Equipment/Environment

• Dispose of soiled dressing and other waste appropriately.

Nurse

• Remove gloves and apron and wash hands.
• Document the care and report any abnormalities.

Points for practice

1. The dressing will need changing if it becomes wet, blood stained or is no longer secure. If it is clean, dry and secure, most local policies will state that it does not need to be changed until the cannula is removed or re-sited.

2. The site should only require cleaning if there is blood present. If pus or exudate is present, the cannula should be removed.

3. If bandaging is required to protect the cannula site (e.g. a confused patient), it will need to be removed regularly to allow visual observation of the site. A light bandage that does not compress the vein should be used.

Removing a peripheral cannula

Preparation

Patient

- Explain the procedure, to gain consent and co-operation.

Equipment/Environment

- The cannula site should be considered as a wound and so should not be exposed unnecessarily or during bed making, dusting, etc.
- Sterile gauze squares.
- Small self-adhesive dressing, or tape and sterile gauze.
- Yellow clinical waste bag.
- Sharps bin.

Procedure

1. Put on gloves.
2. Remove the old dressing, leaving the cannula in situ.
3. Fold a piece of gauze three or four times to create an absorbent pad.
4. Place the folded gauze over the cannula insertion site. Gently withdraw the cannula and immediately apply firm pressure over the insertion site.
5. Continue to apply pressure until the bleeding has stopped (about 3 minutes) to prevent haematoma formation.
6. Apply a small dressing, or tape and a piece of sterile gauze, over the site.

Nurse

- The hands must be washed and dried thoroughly.
- Gloves should be worn. These should be close-fitting to enable manipulation of adhesive dressings and tape.

Post procedure

Patient

- Ensure comfort and advise the patient to report any bleeding or discomfort at the site.

Equipment/Environment

- Discard all waste appropriately.

Nurse

- Remove gloves and apron and wash hands.
- Document removal of cannula and report any abnormalities

Bibliography/Suggested reading

Auty B. Types of infusion pump and their risk. *British Journal of Intensive Care* 1995, **5**(2) supplement: 11–16.

Campbell L. IV-related phlebitis, complications and length of hospital stay – 2. *British Journal of Nursing* 1998, 7:1364–1373.

Campbell T, Lunn D. Intravenous therapy: current practice and nursing concerns. *British Journal of Nursing* 1997, **6**(21):118–122.

Dougherty L. Intravenous cannulation (RCN Continuing Education). *Nursing Standard* 1999, **11**(2):47–51.

Dougherty L, Lamb, J. *Intravenous therapy in nursing practice*. London: Churchill Livingstone; 1999.

Fox N. Managing the risks posed by intravenous therapy. *Nursing Times* 2000, **96**(30):37–39.

Fuller A, Winn C. Selecting equipment for peripheral intravenous cannulation. *Professional Nurse* 1999, **14**(4):233–236.

Given B. Taking the jab out of needles (use of EMLA cream). *Canadian Nurse* 1993, **89**(10):37–40.

Homer LD, Holmes KR. Risks associated with 72 and 96 hour peripheral IV catheter dwell times. *Journal of Intravenous Nursing* 1998, **21**(5):301–305.

Heywood Jones H. Venepuncture using vacuum tubes. In: *Skills update, book 4*. London: Macmillan Magazines; 1995.

Intravenous Nursing Society. Revised intravenous nursing standards of practice. *Journal of Intravenous Nursing* 1998, **21**(15): supplement 1S.

Jackson A. Performing peripheral intravenous cannulation. *Professional Nurse* 1997, **13**(1):21–25.

Lapham R, Agar H. *Drug calculations for nurses: a step by step approach*. London: Arnold; 1995.

Pickstone MA. *A pocketbook for safer IV therapy*. Scitech Educational; 1999.

Royal College of Nursing. *Guidance for nurses giving intravenous therapy*. London: RCN; 1999.

Snelling P, Duffy L. Developing self-directed training for intravenous cannulation. *Professional Nurse* 2002, **18**:137–142.

Thorpe S. *A practical guide to taking blood*. London: Baillière Tindall; 1991.

Wilson J. Preventing infection during IV therapy. *Professional Nurse* 1994, **9**(6):388–392.

Notes

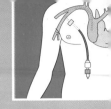

4

Central venous catheters

Preparation

Patient

- Explain the procedure, to gain consent and co-operation.
- The patient should be in a recumbent or semi-recumbent position.

Equipment/Environment

- Ensure warmth, privacy and adequate light.
- Dressing trolley or clean, flat surface adjacent to the patient.
- Sterile dressing pack containing gloves.
- Cleansing solution according to local policy (e.g. chlorhexidine in alcohol).
- Sterile dressing according to policy/protocol **PFP1**.
- Alcohol hand-rub.

Nurse

- The hands must be washed and dried thoroughly.
- An apron should be worn.

Procedure

1. Assemble all equipment at the bedside.
2. Ask/assist the patient into a comfortable recumbent or semi-recumbent position and remove clothing as necessary to expose the site **PFP2**.
3. Open the pack and using the sterile disposal bag as a 'glove', and taking great care not to dislodge the catheter, remove the old dressing and turn the bag inside out to contain it (see page 223). Place the bag in a convenient position to allow easy access.
4. Put on sterile gloves and, if necessary, clean the site according to local policy and allow to dry.
5. Apply the new dressing, making sure that the IV tubing is secured under the dressing, to prevent pulling on the catheter.
6. Remove gloves.

Post procedure

Patient

- Assist the patient as necessary to replace clothing and adopt a comfortable position.
- Instruct the patient to report any pain or discomfort at the site.

Equipment/Environment

- Dispose of all waste appropriately.

Nurse

- Remove apron and wash hands.
- Document the dressing change in the nursing records and report any abnormal findings.

Points for practice

1. Local policy or protocol will determine the type of dressing to be used. Transparent, moisture-permeable dressings are popular because they are occlusive, allow easy visualisation of the site, and provide secure fixing of the intravenous tubing, thus preventing it pulling on the catheter.

2. A catheter for measurement of the central venous pressure (CVP) will be inserted into the internal or external jugular vein or subclavian vein. Central venous catheters for parenteral nutrition or drug administration (and therefore not for CVP measurement) may be inserted into the brachial vein at the antecubital fossa and then advanced until the tip rests in the subclavian vein. This is referred to as a peripherally inserted central catheter (PICC).

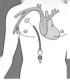

CVP measurement

Preparation

Patient

- Explain the procedure, to gain consent and co-operation.
- The patient should be lying flat or in the same position as adopted for previous CVP measurements.

Equipment/Environment

- CVP manometer with 0.9% sodium chloride infusion. CVP measurements cannot be made with any other solution.

Nurse

- Wash and dry hands thoroughly.
- Check previous CVP measurements and the position of the patient during these measurements (this should be indicated on the chart).

Procedure

1. With the patient lying flat or in the same position as adopted for previous measurements, level the zero point on the manometer with the patient's heart. A spirit level is incorporated into the manometer arm to ensure accurate levelling.
2. A mark should be made at the midaxillary line or sternal angle to indicate the level, so that all subsequent readings are made from the same point.
3. If necessary, turn off any other infusions that may be running through the central venous catheter.
4. With the three-way tap in position 'A' (Figure 4.1), allow the 0.9% sodium chloride infusion to run rapidly for a few seconds to check that the line is patent **PFP1**.
5. Stop the infusion by closing the roller clamp. Adjust the three-way tap on the manometer to position 'B', so that the fluid can go up the column. Gradually open the roller clamp to allow fluid to slowly fill the manometer column until 5–10cm above the previous measurement. Close the roller clamp.
6. Turn the three-way tap to position 'C', so that the line to the infusion bag is closed and the other two lines (to the column and the patient) are open. The fluid in the column will now start to fall, pausing with each respiration, until it equalises with the pressure in the right atrium of the heart. The fluid should continue to rise and fall gently with respiration **PFP2**. This level, which is measured in centimetres of water (cmH$_2$O), is the CVP measurement **PFP3**.
7. Turn the three-way tap back to position 'A', so that the column of fluid is 'off', and reset the infusion to the prescribed rate. Reset any other infusions as appropriate.

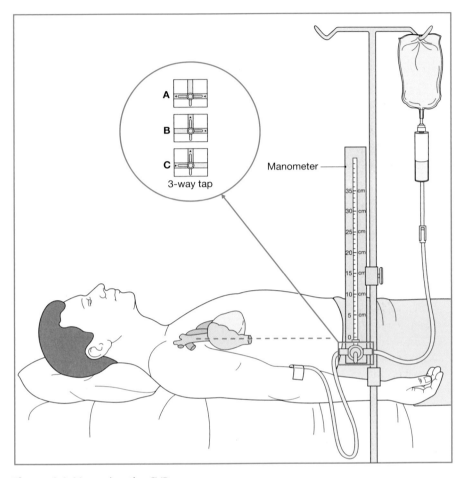

Figure 4.1 Measuring the CVP

Post procedure

Patient

• Assist the patient into a comfortable position.

Equipment/Environment

• Ensure all equipment is secured safely and IV tubing does not touch the floor.

Nurse

• Record the CVP measurement on the appropriate chart. If this is the first measurement, also note the position of the patient and the reference point for readings.
• Report any abnormalities or changes from previous measurements.

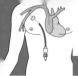

Points for practice

1. If the infusion will not run freely, the CVP measurement will not be accurate. Sometimes, asking the patient to turn their head away from the CVP line or applying gentle traction on the line can help by moving the tip of the catheter away from the wall of the blood vessel. If this makes the infusion run freely, perform the same manoeuvre when measuring the CVP.

2. The fluid in the column should 'swing' with each respiration because of changes in the pressure within the chest. If the fluid falls but does not swing, it may not be an accurate measurement.

3. The normal range for the CVP is 7–12cmH$_2$O if measured at the mid axilla, and 0–7cmH$_2$O if measured at the sternal angle (Woodrow 2002). The reading should be interpreted in conjunction with other signs and the trend (i.e. whether it is rising or falling) is often more important than a single measurement.

Removal of CVP catheter (non-tunnelled)

Preparation

Patient

- Explain the procedure, to ensure understanding and co-operation.
- The patient should be lying flat and slightly head-down if possible **PFP1** .

Equipment/Environment

- Ensure warmth, dignity and privacy.
- Equipment to perform dressing (page 222).
- Sterile air-occlusive dressing **PFP2** .
- Sterile scissors and specimen pot (universal type).
- Cleansing solution according to local policy (e.g. povidone iodine).
- Stitch cutter.
- Sharps bin.
- Alcohol hand-rub or handwashing facilities.

Nurse

- Nurses may remove non-tunnelled CVP catheters **PFP3** . A second nurse may be required to assist during this procedure.
- The hands must be washed and dried thoroughly.
- An apron should be worn.

Procedure

1. Ask/assist the patient to lie flat. Tilt the head of the bed down (about 15°), if the patient's condition will allow. Remove clothing, bedclothes, etc., as necessary to expose the CVP catheter site.
2. Prepare all equipment (see page 222).
3. Turn off the infusion and loosen but do not remove the dressing covering the site.
4. Wash and dry your hands thoroughly or clean them with alcohol hand-rub.
5. Open the dressing pack and using the waste disposal bag as a 'glove' to protect your hand, remove the dressing and turn the bag inside out to contain it (see page 223). Place the bag in a convenient position to allow easy access.
6. Put on the sterile gloves provided in the dressing pack and using a gauze swab and cleansing solution, clean around the insertion site **PFP4** .
7. Using the stitch cutter, cut the stitch holding the catheter in place and make sure it is free of the skin.
8. Maintaining sterility, open the specimen pot and place it in an accessible position.
9. Fold a gauze square three or four times to create an absorbent pad. Holding this in your non-dominant hand, place it over the insertion site, ready to press immediately the catheter is withdrawn.
10. Ask the patient to hold their breath during removal of the catheter. Withdraw the catheter by pulling in a firm, steady movement and press firmly with the gauze pad for several minutes to prevent bleeding and air embolus.

11. Ask an assistant to place the tip of the catheter in the specimen pot and using sterile scissors, cut off the tip (about 5cm) and allow it to fall into the container. Replace the lid **PFP5**.
12. Once the bleeding has stopped, apply the sterile air-occlusive dressing to the site.
13. Remove gloves.

Post procedure

Patient

• Return the bed to the horizontal position and ask the patient to remain supine for 15–30 minutes following removal.

Equipment/Environment

• Dispose of all clinical waste and sharps appropriately.

Nurse

• Wash and dry hands thoroughly.
• Label the specimen container and with the appropriate request form, send for bacteriological examination.
• Document CVP removal in the nursing records.

Points for practice

1. There is a significant risk of air embolism during and after the removal of a CVP catheter (Menim et al 1992). Placing the patient in a supine, head-down position reduces this by increasing the intrathoracic pressure, making it less likely for air to be drawn in during inspiration. Forceful inspiration following a cough may facilitate entry of air.

2. An air-occlusive dressing must be used to reduce the risk of air entry leading to air embolus following removal of the catheter (Menim et al 1992).

3. Local policy may dictate that only nurses who have undergone additional training may remove CVP catheters. Tunnelled catheters must be removed by medical staff and often require surgical removal.

4. The site must be cleaned before removal of the catheter, to prevent contamination of the tip during withdrawal, which would lead to an inaccurate bacteriological assessment.

5. Most hospital protocols require the tip of the catheter to be sent for bacterial examination following removal. If no assistance is available, place the catheter on the trolley so that the tip is resting on a corner of the sterile field, to prevent contamination. Once the dressing is securely in place, cut the tip off as described.

Principles

Hickman and Groshong lines are types of central venous catheters made of special hypoallergenic material that allow them to remain in situ for many months. They are often used for patients who require regular, but intermittent, intravenous therapy, such as those receiving chemotherapy or total parenteral nutrition (TPN). As with all central venous catheters, there is a high risk of infection, especially with patients who are immunosuppressed and/or receiving chemotherapy, and therefore asepsis is vital. In order to reduce the risk of infection, long-term catheters are tunnelled under the skin (Figure 4.2). This means that the insertion site through the skin, which is very vulnerable to infection, is well away from the point of entry into the blood vessel, thus reducing the risk of septicaemia.

Care of the site

Care of long-term catheters is often undertaken at home by patients or carers or by the district nurse. The dressing over the cannula site should be changed twice weekly until the tissue around the Dacron cuff has become fibrosed. This cuff aids catheter security (preventing accidental dislodgement) and acts as a barrier to the movement of micro-organisms along the catheter. Long-term care varies considerably from hospital to hospital, but covering the site is not usually necessary once the site has healed, except when there is a risk of it getting wet, e.g. in the shower.

Immersion of the site is not recommended, but splashing, as in the shower, is usually no problem. Bathing in a public pool and water sports are not recommended because of the risk of infection from the water. In order to remain patent, the catheter must be flushed at regular intervals to prevent clotting. Most hospitals recommend the use of heparinised saline two to three times per week, but recommended practices vary in both frequency and the solution used.

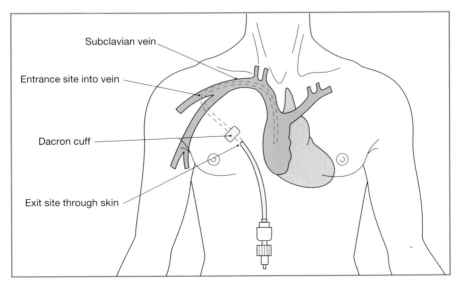

Figure 4.2 Tunnelled long-term catheter

Total parenteral nutrition

Total parenteral nutrition (TPN) is most commonly administered via a central venous catheter, which because of the irritant nature of the high dextrose solution, is the route of choice. Tunnelled CVP catheters are recommended for TPN; however, administration via a peripheral line is used in some situations. The administration set being used for TPN must be changed every 24 hours with each new bag. The bags of feed must be stored in a designated refrigerator and removed 2 hours prior to administration (1 hour may be sufficient in hot weather). If there are no lipids in the bag, it must be covered to prevent degradation of the vitamins by exposure to light.

The line must be flushed with 0.9% sodium chloride containing heparin before commencing and after completion of a feed. The CVP catheter being used for TPN must not be used for measurement or drug administration because any interruption in the closed system increases the risk of infection. There is also a high risk of incompatibility with medicines.

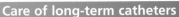

Bibliography/Suggested reading

Cornock M. Making sense of central venous pressure (CVP). *Nursing Times* 1996, **92**(40):38–39.

Cornock M. Making sense of central venous catheters. *Nursing Times* 1996, **92**(49):30–31.

Dougherty L, Lamb J. *Intravenous therapy in nursing practice*. London: Churchill Livingstone; 1999.

Gabriel J. Care and management of peripherally inserted central catheters. *British Journal of Nursing* 1996, **5**(10): 594–599.

Henry L. Parenteral nutrition. *Professional Nurse* 1997, **13**(1):39–42.

Mennim P, Coyle C, Taylor J. Venous air embolism associated with removal of central venous catheter. *British Medical Journal* 1992, **305**:171–172.

Perry C, Leaper D. Care of central venous line exit sites. *Journal of Wound Care* 1994, **3**(6):279–282.

Pratt R. Preventing infections associated with central venous catheters. *Nursing Times* 2001, **97**(15):36–39.

Simcock L. The use of central venous catheters for IV therapy. *Nursing Times* 2001, **97**(18):34–35.

Simcock L. Central venous catheters: some common clinical questions. *Nursing Times* 2001, **97**(19):34–35.

Todd J. Peripherally inserted central catheters. *Professional Nurse* 1998, **13**(5):297–302.

Woodrow P. Central venous catheters and central venous pressure. *Nursing Standard* 2002, **16**(26):45–52.

Notes

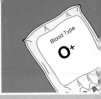

5

Blood transfusion

Principles

- It is vital that blood for transfusion is checked carefully to ensure that the correct blood is administered to the correct patient. Fatal consequences can ensue if the incorrect blood is given.
- Adverse reactions most commonly occur within 10–15 minutes of commencing transfusion and so it is vital that nurses continually observe the patient during this time. The frequency of observations after that time will vary according to local policy.
- Until relatively recently, blood was always checked by two nurses, one of whom had to be a registered nurse and many local policies require this. However, guidance from the British Committee for Standards in Haematology (BCSH 1999) now recommends that one registered nurse carry out the checking procedure. Whatever the policy, it is vital that all checking is carried out at the bedside.
- All patients receiving a blood transfusion must be wearing an identification name band.

Storage of blood

- Blood must be stored in a special refrigerator at 2–6°C to prevent contaminants reproducing. It must not be kept in a ward refrigerator.
- Blood for transfusion should be collected from the blood transfusion department or special refrigerator no longer than 30 minutes before it is required. This is because pathogens grow extremely quickly in blood at room temperature. If the transfusion has not commenced within this time, the blood bank must be informed and the blood may need to be discarded.
- If the blood is stored in a special 'blood carrier' this time may be extended (see local policy).

Blood bag

- The bag should be checked to ensure that it is not leaking or wet and that there is no turbidity or discoloration.
- The bag must have a compatibility label attached (Figure 5.1).
- Drugs must never be added to blood.
- Blood must never be warmed by placing it in hot water or in a microwave. Direct heat will cause blood to haemolyse (Bradbury & Cruickshank 2000). If warming is required, a blood warmer should be used (see below and page 94).

Administration

- A special blood administration set that incorporates a filter chamber must be used. An additional in-line filter may be required where multiple units of blood are to be administered. Refer to local policy.
- Electronic infusion pumps must not be used as the red blood cells may be damaged during infusion.
- There is no evidence that warming the blood is beneficial if it is administered slowly, but if rapid transfusion of large volumes is required (> 50ml/kg/hour) or blood is being administered via a central venous catheter, a blood warmer should be used (Bradbury & Cruickshank 2000).

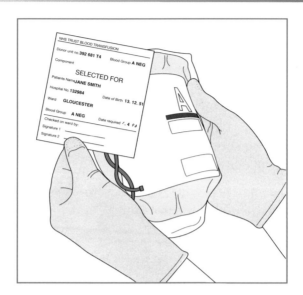

Figure 5.1 Blood bag with compatibility label

Documentation

- All documentation must be checked during the checking process. For example, it is insufficient merely to look at the patient's name band to confirm the name and hospital number, as the details may not be correct. The medical case notes, the blood transfusion compatibility report form, the compatibility label and the prescription chart must also be checked (see checking procedure below).

Blood transfusion checking procedure

1. Check the patient's identity

- All checking must take place at the bedside.
- Where possible, positively identify patients by asking them to state their full name and date of birth. Check that these match the name band.

2. Check the patient's surname, first names, sex, date of birth, hospital number, blood group and rhesus factor on:

- Patient's name band.
- Blood transfusion compatibility report form.
- Compatibility label attached to the bag.
- Medical case notes.
- Intravenous (IV) fluid prescription chart.

3. Check the expiry date of the unit of blood (and time if applicable, e.g. platelets) on:

- Compatibility label on the bag.
- Blood bag.

4. Check the blood group and unit number on:

- Blood transfusion compatibility report form.
- Compatibility label on the bag.

5. Check any special requirements

- The unit of blood must comply with the prescription chart (e.g. gamma irradiated).

6. Record the unit number of the blood on:

- The IV fluid prescription chart.

7. Record the date and time and signature of the nurse(s) on:

- Blood transfusion compatibility report form.
- Compatibility label.
- IV fluid prescription chart.

If any discrepancies are noted, the blood must not be transfused, the blood bank must be informed, and the blood and blood transfusion compatibility form returned.

Preparation

Patient
- Explain the procedure, to gain consent and co-operation (the patient will be closely observed throughout the transfusion).
- The patient must be wearing a name band.
- Advise the patient not to leave the ward during the transfusion (in many instances patients will be confined to bed).

Equipment/Environment
- Blood administration set **PFP1** .
- Clinical thermometer and watch.
- Sphygmomanometer and stethoscope.
- Observation chart (temperature, pulse, respiration and blood pressure).
- Fluid balance chart.
- IV prescription chart.
- IV hydrocortisone and chlorpheniramine should be available on the ward (in case of allergic reactions).

Nurse
- Wash and dry hands thoroughly.
- Gloves and an apron should be worn.

Procedure

1. At the bedside, check the blood as described on page 89. Blood must be checked by a registered nurse, before transfusion. Some local policies will require two nurses to check (see page 88).
2. Prepare the infusion as described on page 61 **PFP2** .
3. Record baseline observations of temperature, pulse, respiration and blood pressure immediately prior to commencement of the transfusion.
4. Record the temperature, pulse, respiration and blood pressure again 15 minutes after commencement of the transfusion. These observations should be repeated at regular intervals throughout the transfusion according to local policy **PFP3** and again at the end of the transfusion.
5. Observe the urine output for volume and colour throughout the transfusion **PFP4** .
6. Observe for and encourage the patient to report any of the following reactions **PFP5** :
   - Facial flushing.
   - A rash on the chest or abdomen.
   - Pain or inflammation at the cannula site.
   - Circulatory overload (rising pulse and respiration rates).
   - Headaches.
   - Feeling hot and flushed or shivering.
   - Chest or abdominal pain, or pain in the extremities.
   - Lumbar or loin pain.
   - Oedema of the eyes or face.

- Laryngeal swelling and/or dyspnoea or 'bubbly' respiration.
- Rigors.
- Oliguria.
7. The transfusion should be stopped and medical staff informed if:
   - There is a rise in temperature of greater than 1°C.
   - There is a significant rise or fall in blood pressure.
   - There is a significant rise in pulse rate.
   - Any of the other reactions occur.
8. If the transfusion continues for more than 12 hours, the administration set should be changed every 12 hours.
9. The blood transfusion compatibility form must be readily available throughout the transfusion.

Post procedure

Patient

- Ensure the patient is comfortable.
- Instruct the patient to observe for and report any reaction or complications.

Equipment/Environment

- Replace equipment and discard waste appropriately.
- The empty blood bags should be kept on the ward or returned to the blood transfusion department according to local policy **PFP6** .
- Change the administration set every 12 hours during the transfusion and at the end of the transfusion if an IV infusion is to follow.

Nurse

- Document the blood transfusion in the nursing records.
- Secure the blood transfusion compatibility report form in the medical notes.
- Report any abnormalities or complications.

Points for practice

1. A special administration set must be used for blood transfusions. This has an additional chamber above the drip chamber, which contains a filter. This filters out debris (platelets and white cells) (see Figure 3.4B, page 63).

2. Platelet administration requires a special administration set with no filter. Platelets must be administered rapidly (20–30 minutes) as soon as they are available.

3. Observations during blood transfusion should be recorded separately from routine observations. Trust policies regarding the frequency of the observations required during blood transfusion may vary, but most suggest that the temperature, pulse, respiration rate and blood pressure should be recorded before the start of the transfusion, 15 minutes after commencement, and again at the end of the transfusion. Each unit of blood should be regarded as a new transfusion. The first 15 minutes of a transfusion is the period when severe reactions most commonly occur (Bradbury & Cruickshank 2000).

4. The urine output should be monitored to detect pyrogenic, antibody and allergic reactions, infection and circulatory overload.

5. If an adverse reaction occurs, the transfusion must be stopped immediately and the medical staff informed. The administration set should be changed and venous access maintained by an infusion of 0.9% sodium chloride. The patient's temperature, pulse, respiration rate and blood pressure and the colour and volume of urine should be monitored.

6. The used blood bags are kept for at least 2 days following transfusion in case there is a delayed reaction to the blood. The procedure for storage and return of these to the blood transfusion department will vary from hospital to hospital.

Use of blood filters

- A blood administration set that includes a 170μm filter chamber is all that is required for most blood transfusions.
- Some patients who are receiving multiple blood transfusions or who have had febrile reactions in response to previous transfusions may require an additional filter. These are fine-mesh filters that are placed between the blood bag and the administration set in order to remove microaggregates (e.g. fibrin and clots) formed during storage. The same filter can be used for up to four units of blood. They are usually supplied with the blood when collected from the blood transfusion department.

Use of blood warmers

- When rapid transfusion or transfusion via a CVP line is necessary, blood may be warmed during administration using a blood warmer. Blood must never be warmed by heating the bag in hot water, on a radiator or in a microwave, as direct heat can cause blood to haemolyse. The design of blood warmers will vary, but most incorporate a 'zig-zag' tube or coil through which the blood passes over a heater element and is warmed before reaching the patient.

Bibliography/Suggested reading

Atterbury C, Wilkinson J. Blood transfusion. *Nursing Standard* 2000, **14**(34):47–52.

BCSH. The administration of blood and blood products and the management of transfused patients. *Transfusion Medicine* 1999, 9:227–238.

Bradbury M, Cruickshank J. Blood transfusion: crucial steps in maintaining safe practice. *British Journal of Nursing* 2000, 9(3):134–138.

Campbell J. Blood groups and transfusions. *Professional Nurse* 1996, **12**(1):39–40, 43–44.

Contreras M, DeSilva M. Preventing incompatible transfusions. *British Medical Journal* 1994, **308**:1180–1181.

Department of Health. *Better blood transfusions.* www.doh.gov.uk/blood/bbt.htm

Godfrey K. In the bag. *Nursing Times* 2000, 96(14):26–27.

Higgins C. Blood transfusion: risks and benefits. *British Journal of Nursing* 1994, 3(19):986–991.

McKenna C. Blood minded. *Nursing Times* 2000, **96**(14):27–28.

Shamash J. Blood counts. *Nursing Times* 2002, **98**(45):23–26.

SHOT (serious hazards of transfusion) Annual report 1999–2000. Manchester: SHOT, 2001.

Notes

6

Nutrition and hydration

Principles

Good nutrition is essential not only to promote health and well-being but also to aid recovery from trauma, surgery or disease. Yet there is growing evidence that malnutrition is common among hospital patients. Many hospital patients do not receive enough food and in some wards up to 60% do not eat enough calories or protein (Bond 1997). Poor nutritional status is known to be associated with delayed recovery and adverse outcomes of illness and injury (Ward & Rollins 1999). Nurses have an important role to play in the prevention of malnutrition. Primarily they should identify those at risk of malnutrition and plan care to meet their needs. In addition they have a role in ensuring those who are initially well-nourished do not become malnourished whilst in hospital. Appropriate and ongoing assessment is a key factor.

Nutritional assessment tools

Most hospitals have developed a tool to assist in nutritional assessment and the identification of those at risk. One monitoring tool for patients over 18 years of age that is often used in conjunction with a nutritional assessment tool, is Body Mass Index (BMI). If the patient is unable to stand, arm span can be used instead of height. This is measured by extending both arms sideways from the body at shoulder height and measuring the distance between the tips of the middle fingers. BMI is calculated by dividing the weight in kilograms (kg) by the height in metres squared (see below). A BMI of 20–24.9 indicates an average or desirable weight. A BMI of greater than 30 is classified as obese and greater than 40 as grossly obese. Patients with a BMI of less than 20 may show signs of malnutrition. It is important to note however that patients who are overweight or obese can also be malnourished.

$$BM1 = \frac{\text{weight in Kg}}{(\text{height in metres})^2} \quad \text{e.g.} \quad \frac{60}{1.69 \times 1.69} = 20.01$$

In addition to the BMI, most nutritional assessment tools will incorporate consideration of the following factors, which are known to increase the risk of malnutrition.

- **Mental condition** – any deterioration in mental state or conscious level is likely to affect the patient's desire and ability to eat and drink independently and so will increase the risk of malnutrition. This includes patients who may be depressed, lethargic or apathetic.
- **Weight** – it is important to note whether there has been any recent weight loss particularly if it is unintentional. This may be apparent from loose-fitting clothes, rings or dentures. Patients who appear thin or emaciated are at an increased risk of malnutrition. Less than 5% weight loss in 6 months is not significant. Between 5–9% is only significant if the patient is already malnourished. Between 10–20% is clinically significant and requires intervention, and more than 20% weight loss may require long-term support.
- **Appetite** – patients who are able to maintain their usual appetite and eating habits are less likely to be at risk than those who have a poor appetite or

refuse meals and drinks. It is important to check whether the patient has altered their eating habits recently.

- **Functioning of the gastrointestinal tract** – the presence of diarrhoea or constipation is likely to affect the desire to eat and drink and may also lead to malabsorption. Nausea and vomiting are also likely to result in a reduced nutritional intake. Patients who are unable to take oral food or fluids following surgery involving the gastrointestinal tract or who have conditions affecting it, such as intestinal obstruction, will be at high risk.
- **Skin and pressure ulcers** – dry and scaling skin may be an indication of dehydration and possibly related malnourishment. The existence of pressure ulcers is significant and is often included on nutritional assessment tools. Pressure ulcers are often associated with poor nutrition and healing pressure ulcers requires increased nutritional intake.
- **Dexterity** – it is important to assess whether patients have the manual dexterity to feed themselves.
- **Other factors** – a number of conditions will affect the ability to eat and so will increase the risk of developing malnutrition. These include:
  - neurological conditions, especially those affecting co-ordination or mental state
  - difficulty swallowing (e.g. after stroke) and malabsorption
  - surgery or major trauma
  - malignant disease and chronic conditions such as chronic obstructive pulmonary disease
  - reduced mobility or confinement to bed
  - bereavement, depression or other mental ill health.

As with tools designed to identify patients at risk of developing pressure ulcers, most nutritional assessment tools involve a scoring system that allocates a score for each of the possible contributing factors. The total score will indicate whether the patient is at risk; appropriate measures can then be taken. Whether a high score indicates a high or a low risk will vary between different assessment tools. Patients identified as high risk should be referred to a dietician. Patients must be assessed within 24 hours of admission. The frequency of further assessments should be determined by the result of the initial assessment. For example if a patient is well nourished on admission to hospital then weekly reassessment is adequate. However if the nutritional assessment score indicates at-risk then reassessment may need to be within 48 hours.

Preparation

Patient

- Establish what the patient would like to eat and drink and whether there are any dietary restrictions.
- Ensure the patient is comfortable, i.e. has an empty bladder, clean hands, clean mouth and, if applicable, clean dentures.
- Ask/assist the patient to sit upright if their condition allows.
- Check the patient is able to swallow, to prevent choking and aspiration into the lungs.

Equipment/Environment

- Remove any offensive materials from the patient's table/eating area, e.g. sputum pot, urinals, etc.
- Clear a space for the tray.
- Position a chair beside the bed for the nurse.

Nurse

- Wash and dry hands thoroughly.
- Put on apron (appropriate colour if applicable) **PFP1** .

Procedure

1. Aim to make the mealtime a pleasant experience for the patient.
2. Obtain the correct food and drink, cutlery and napkin.
3. Set the meal out in a pleasing manner to tempt the appetite.
4. Take the tray to the bedside, and if the patient is unable to see the food, describe the meal **PFP2** .
5. Cut up the food if necessary.
6. Protect the patient's clothing with a napkin or paper towel.
7. Sit down so that a more relaxed approach is conveyed to the patient (Figure 6.1).
8. Tailor the speed and manner in which food/drink is offered according to the patient's needs/wishes. It should not be hurried **PFP3,4** .
9. Allow the patient time to chew and swallow the food before presenting the next mouthful. Adjust the size of the mouthful to suit the patient.
10. Avoid asking questions while the patient is eating.
11. Respect the patient's dignity and use the napkin to remove dribbles of food or drink that may run down the chin.
12. When giving a drink, tip the cup/glass very gently so that the flow is controlled. Care should be taken with hot drinks, particularly if using a polystyrene cup, as it is difficult to judge the temperature of the liquid inside.
13. Encourage the patient to eat and drink if necessary, but do not press patients once they have indicated that they have had sufficient. Small amounts taken more frequently may be more successful.

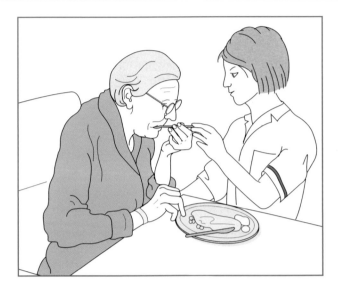

Figure 6.1 Feeding the patient

Post procedure

Patient

- Assist the patient to meet hygiene needs (mouth, teeth and hands) as necessary.

Equipment/Environment

- Remove unwanted food, crockery and cutlery.
- Wipe up any spillages on the table or locker.
- Restore the patient's environment, i.e. put a glass of water and the patient's belongings back within easy reach.

Nurse

- Remove apron and wash hands.
- Complete relevant documentation, i.e. fluid balance and/or food chart.
- Report any abnormal occurrences, e.g. vomiting, food refusal.

Points for practice

1. In some hospitals, different-coloured aprons are used for activities such as serving meals, washing patients and doing dressings.

2. If supervising the patient rather than feeding them, place all food and drink within easy reach of the patient. If the patient is visually impaired, 'clock' instructions may help them locate different foods, e.g. meat is at 12 o'clock, potatoes are at 5 o'clock, etc.

3. Always check any particular cultural practices related to eating and drinking. For example, where possible, a Muslim patient should be fed with the right hand as the left hand is considered 'dirty'.

4. If the patient is only able to use one hand, a plate guard and non-slip mat may help. If they are unable to grip ordinary cutlery, large-handled cutlery can usually be obtained from the occupational therapy department.

Preparation

Patient

- Respond promptly to calls for assistance.

Equipment/Environment

- Draw screens if time permits, to ensure privacy.
- Provide vomit bowl (usually disposable).
- Provide tissues or paper towels.

Nurse

- Put on apron and gloves (if time).

Procedure

1. If possible, remove the patient's dentures (where applicable) and store them safely.
2. Ask/assist the patient to sit forward, or if lying down or semi-conscious, place in the lateral position to reduce the risk of aspiration.
3. Support the patient's forehead.
4. Encourage the patient to breathe more deeply if possible.
5. Provide tissues and promote comfort and dignity by wiping the patient's mouth if the patient is too weak or distressed to do this unaided.
6. Never leave the patient without a vomit bowl – get a clean one before removing the used one, even if the patient feels the episode has passed.

Post procedure

Patient

- Offer a mouthwash or perform mouth care if the patient is too weak.
- Offer the patient a bowl for face and hand-washing.

Equipment/Environment

- Cover the vomit bowl before removing it from the bedside.
- Identify the type of vomit and measure the amount **PFP1,2** .
- Save the vomit for inspection if necessary (e.g. haematemesis) **PFP3** .

Nurse

- If appropriate, administer anti-emetic drugs as prescribed and monitor the effect **PFP4** .
- Document the vomiting episode, making a note of nausea, frequency, amount and whether related to food.
- Report if vomiting is a new occurrence or if the vomiting has altered in any way.
- Ascertain the cause of vomiting if possible, and take appropriate action.

Points for practice

1. When observing vomit you should note the amount, frequency, whether accompanied by pain or nausea and whether associated with any medication (e.g. analgesic), surgery, type of food or other cause. Also note whether it is projectile vomit (vomit that is emitted with force).

2. The vomit may contain undigested food or be watery (gastric juices only) or a green/brown fluid (indicates presence of bile). If the vomit is brown and foul (faecal) smelling, this may indicate that there is an obstruction in the large intestine.

3. The term haematemesis means blood in the vomit. If this is bright red, it indicates fresh blood from the stomach or upper gastrointestinal tract; if it is dark brown and 'coffee ground' in appearance, this is older blood that has been partially digested.

4. Post-operative nausea and vomiting causes distress and suffering for many surgical patients. The prophylactic administration of prescribed anti-emetic medication can greatly reduce this.

Preparation

Patient

- Explain the procedure, to gain consent and co-operation.
- Patients receiving subcutaneous fluids are often older adults and are sometimes confused. A second nurse may be necessary to comfort the patient **PFP1**

Equipment/Environment

- Prescribed fluid and additive (if applicable) **PFP2**.
- Standard administration set.
- Small (21 G) 'butterfly'-type intravenous cannula.
- Transparent occlusive dressing (approximately 10 cm × 10 cm).

Nurse

- Wash and dry hands thoroughly and put on gloves.
- Only registered nurses may insert the cannula and subcutaneous infusions must be checked by a registered nurse.

Procedure

1. Check the prescribed fluid and prime the administration set to expel all air (see page 61).
2. At the bedside, ask/assist the patient to move into a suitable position to allow access to the site **PFP3**. Check the patient's name band against the prescription.
3. Clean the skin with an alcohol-impregnated swab and allow to dry.
4. Maintaining asepsis, remove the protective cover from the cannula and hold it with the beveled edge facing upwards. Pinch the skin up slightly and insert the needle into the subcutaneous tissue at an angle of 45° (Figure 6.2). If blood appears in the tubing, withdraw the cannula and repeat the process at another site using a new cannula.

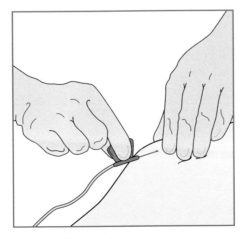

Figure 6.2 Inserting the butterfly cannula

5. Cover the area with the transparent dressing.
6. Set the infusion to the prescribed rate (see page 66).

Post procedure

Patient

- Ensure the patient is comfortable.
- Observe the cannula site for redness, swelling or discomfort.
- Change the infusion site regularly, according to local policy **PFP4** .

Equipment/Environment

- Dispose of all clinical waste appropriately.

Nurse

- Document the subcutaneous infusion in the nursing records.
- Record/monitor fluid balance according to local policy.

Points for practice

1. Subcutaneous fluids are most commonly used for older adults with dehydration where there is no indication for intravenous fluids.

2. Dextrose saline or 0.9% sodium chloride are the solutions most commonly administered subcutaneously. An enzyme (hyaluronidase), which causes more rapid diffusion of the fluid by reducing normal interstitial barriers, may be prescribed. This may be injected into the site via the cannula prior to commencement of the infusion, or added to the infusion bag.

3. Any site with sufficient subcutaneous tissue may be used. The nurse should consider patient comfort and mobility, ease of access and skin condition when choosing the site. The abdomen and thighs are commonly used although the area over the scapula and anterior chest wall are ideal.

4. Ideally the infusion site should be changed after 2L of fluid or every 24 hours although every 48 hours has been suggested as adequate (Mansfield 1998).

Preparation

Patient

- Explain the procedure, to gain consent and co-operation.
- Draw screens to ensure privacy.
- Ensure the patient is comfortable – sitting upright if possible **PFP1** .
- Protect the patient's clothing with a towel.

Equipment/Environment

- Prepare space at the bedside.
- Nasogastric tube of appropriate size and type (e.g. Ryles type, fine bore).
- Lubricant (water-soluble jelly, or water).
- pH strips
- Receiver or vomit bowl.
- A 10ml syringe.
- Two small gallipots.
- Tape, tissues, yellow waste bag.

Nurse

- Wash and dry hands thoroughly.
- Put on apron and gloves.

Procedure

1. Take the equipment to the bedside.
2. Estimate the length of tube to be inserted by measuring the distance from the patient's nose to the tip of the ear lobe and then to the xiphisternum, and make a note of where this is on the tube (Figure 6.3) **PFP2** .
3. Ask/assist the patient to remove dentures and to clear nasal passages by blowing the nose. Select the best nostril (not tender, no deviated septum, etc.).
4. Encourage the patient to relax as much as possible and to breathe steadily.
5. Lubricate the tip of the tube.
6. Pass the tube gently into the nostril and pass backwards (not upwards) along the floor of the nose to the nasopharynx. (If a blockage is felt, change to the other nostril.)
7. Pause to allow the patient to draw breath and recover.
8. Ask the patient to breathe through their mouth and swallow. As the patient swallows, and while keeping the head level, gently advance the tube. A sip of water may help the patient 'swallow' the tube.
9. When the tube has reached the measured distance, check it is in the stomach by one or more of the following methods.
   - Aspirating a small amount of stomach contents from the tube with a 10ml syringe. Apply aspirate to a pH strip, leave for 1 minute and then compare to colour bars to get a reading. A pH of less than 4 confirms gastric placement **PFP3** .

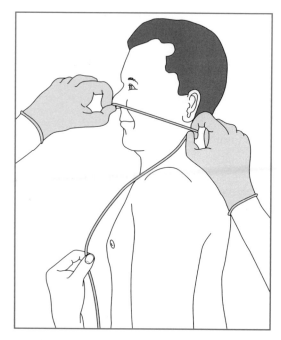

Figure 6.3 Measuring the length of tube to be inserted

- If unable to obtain any aspirate or the pH is greater than 4, the position of the tube should be confirmed by X-ray. X-ray should be used to confirm the position of the tube in all unconscious patients.
10. Secure the tube ensuring that friction or pressure on the tip of the nose is avoided and the patient's vision is not obstructed.

Post procedure

Patient

- Ensure the patient is comfortable.

Equipment/Environment

- Clear away the equipment.
- Dispose of waste appropriately.
- If a fine-bore tube has been used, remove the guidewire following X-ray **PFP4**.

Nurse

- Remove gloves and apron and wash hands.
- Document nasogastric tube insertion and report any abnormal findings.

Points for practice

1. Insertion of the nasogastric tube may be for feeding or for gastric aspiration. The upright position is best for nasogastric tube insertion; if this is not possible, the patient should be lying on one side.

2. Having measured the tube, make a note of how much will remain outside the nose. The tube may have markings on it to facilitate this. It is important to measure the tube to ensure that it does not pass through the stomach and into the duodenum.

3. Changes to the pH strip may not occur in some clinical conditions (e.g. pernicious anaemia or previous gastrectomy) or if the patient is receiving H_2-receptor antagonists (which decrease the secretion of gastric acid) or if the tube has passed through the pylorus. Flushing the tube with 20ml of air prior to obtaining aspirate will ensure removal of any nasopharyngeal secretions that have entered the tube during insertion.

4. If a fine-bore tube has been inserted, the guide wire should be left in position until an X-ray has confirmed the position of the tube in the stomach. The guide wire is then removed by holding the tube at the nose with one hand and pulling the wire out with the other. Do not reinsert the guide wire after removal, as there is a risk of perforation of the oesophageal or stomach wall.

Preparation

Patient

- Explain the procedure, to gain consent and co-operation.
- Ensure the patient is comfortable and sitting upright if condition permits.

Equipment/Environment

- Nasogastric feeding pump, or reservoir bottle or bag if a gravity method is being used.
- Prescribed nasogastric feed plus enteral administration set.
- Syringe and sterile water **PFP1**.
- Syringe, gallipot and pH strips to check tube position **PFP2**.

Nurse

- Wash and dry hands thoroughly.
- Put on apron.

Procedure

1. Take the equipment to the bedside.
2. Check the nasogastric tube is in the stomach aspirating a small amount of stomach contents from the tube with a syringe. Apply aspirate to a pH strip, leave for 1 minute and then compare to colour bars to get a reading. A pH of less than 4 confirms gastric placement (see page 109).
3. Remove the cap of the feed bottle and attach the administration set according to the manufacturer's instructions. If a separate reservoir is being used, pour the feed into the bag/reservoir and attach the administration set. (Sterile water may be given via this method.)
4. Allow the feed to run through the tubing to expel all air and then close the roller clamp.
5. Connect the administration set to the nasogastric tube securely.
6. If using a pump, insert the administration set according to the manufacturer's instructions and open the roller clamp. Switch the pump on (Figure 6.4), set it to the prescribed rate and press 'start'. If a gravity method is being used, adjust the roller clamp until the prescribed flow rate is achieved.

Post procedure

Patient

- Ensure the patient is comfortable and observe for signs of nausea, gastric reflux or dyspnoea.
- Attend to the patient's hygiene (mouth, lips and nostrils) as necessary.
- Observe for diarrhoea or constipation.

Equipment/Environment

- Clear away the equipment and wipe up any spillages.

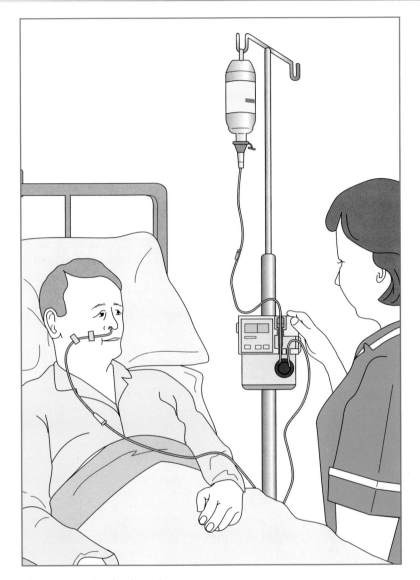

Figure 6.4 Nasogastric feeding via a pump

- When the feed has finished, detach the bottle from the administration set and flush the nasogastric tube with 20–30ml of sterile water to prevent stasis of feed in the tube **PFP3**.
- Change the administration set every 24 hours. Attach label indicating date and time set up.

Nurse

- Remove apron and wash hands.
- Record the feed on the fluid balance chart and other relevant documentation.
- Report any complications.

Points for practice

1. The size of syringe required to aspirate the tube will vary. If a fine-bore tube is used, a 10ml syringe will be adequate. However, if a Ryles-type (large-bore) tube is used, it will not be possible to attach an ordinary syringe: a 50ml catheter-tip syringe will be necessary. When aspirating, it is important to avoid creating too much suction as being sucked against the end of the tube may damage the gastric mucosa.

2. It is vital to check the position of the tube prior to each feed. If a fine-bore tube is used, the patient may not always show signs of distress if the tube (and subsequently nasogastric feed) enters the lungs.

3. If a second bottle of feed is due to commence, ensure that the first does not empty completely, allowing air to enter the administration set. If this does happen, the set will need to be disconnected and primed again before the second feed can commence.

Principles

- The site should be treated as a wound after insertion of a percutaneous endoscopic gastrostomy (PEG) tube. Although local practices may vary, most policies recommend that the site is cleaned with sterile 0.9% sodium chloride, sprayed with an iodine-based powder spray, and a sterile self-adhesive gauze dressing applied.
- The dressing should be changed twice weekly unless the stoma is discharging, in which case it should be changed daily. When the area has healed, no dressing is necessary.
- The site should be observed for signs of inflammation, excoriation and gastric leakage, and the patient's temperature and pulse rate should be monitored for 7 days.
- Once the site has healed, the guard surrounding the tube (Figure 6.5) should be lifted up daily and slid round the tube so that the area can be washed with warm soapy water and then dried thoroughly. The tube should then be rotated, to prevent necrosis caused by pressure from the balloon inside the stomach. The guard is then replaced.
- The patient is able to bathe or shower providing the gastrostomy tube is closed. The site should be dried thoroughly afterwards.

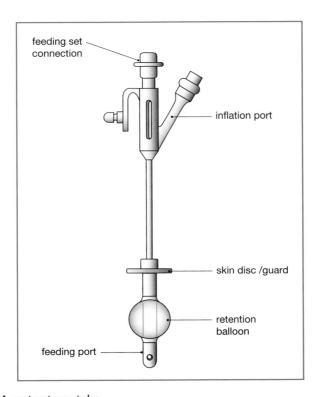

feeding set connection

inflation port

skin disc /guard

retention balloon

feeding port

Figure 6.5 A gastrostomy tube

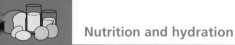
- The gastrostomy tube is not usually used on the day of insertion (but can be used within 6–12 hours if bowel sounds are present) and a short course of antibiotics (often intravenously) is usually prescribed. When bowel sounds are established, feeding may commence. The tube should be flushed with 25–30ml of sterile water before and after feeds and the administration of drugs.

Preparation

Patient

- Explain the procedure, to gain consent and co-operation PFP1,2 .
- It is advisable for the patient to be sitting up (unless the feed is given very slowly).
- Bowel sounds should be present PFP3 .

Equipment/Environment

- Prescription chart and prescribed feed.
- Enteral feed administration set.
- Syringe (to flush tube).
- Water (sterile).
- Enteral feed pump.
- Infusion stand.
- Fluid balance chart.

Nurse

- Wash and dry hands thoroughly.
- Put on apron.

Procedure

1. Take the equipment and the feed to the bedside and check the patient's name band.
2. Remove the cap of the feed bottle.
3. Maintaining asepsis, open the enteral feed administration set, attach it to the bottle according to the manufacturer's instructions, and close the flow control roller clamp PFP4 .
4. Attach the hanger to the feed container and hang the feed container on the infusion stand.
5. Open the roller clamp on the administration set, allow the feed to run through to expel all air and then close the clamp. The plastic cap on the end of the administration set should remain in place so that the tube remains sterile.
6. Using the syringe, draw up the water (25–30ml depending on local policy) and flush the tube PFP5 .
7. Insert the administration set into the pump according to the manufacturer's instructions, remove the plastic cap at the distal end of it and attach it to the PEG tube.
8. Open the roller clamp and turn on the pump.
9. Set the flow rate as prescribed (e.g. 125ml per hour) and start the pump.
10. Check that the feed is running and is not leaking at the connection with the PEG tube and that the tube is not kinked or blocked.

Post procedure

Patient

- Ensure the patient is comfortable. Observe PEG site regularly **PFP6**.
- Return regularly, to check the feed is running satisfactorily.
- Observe the patient for nausea, vomiting or diarrhoea.

Equipment/Environment

- Clear away equipment and wipe up any spillages, especially on the pump.
- On completion of the feed, disconnect the administration set and flush the tube with sterile water according to local policy **PFP7**.
- The pump usually has alarms to indicate when the feed has finished or if the tube has become blocked or kinked.
- If there are no alarms, extra checking is required.

Nurse

- Remove apron and wash hands.
- Document the type of feed, time started, rate of flow and volume of water used to flush the tube.

Points for practice

1. As eating and drinking are social activities as well as physical necessities, it is important to try and make PEG/gastrostomy feeds as pleasant and 'normal' as possible, e.g. if the feed is not continuous, by administering the feed when others are eating their meals.

2. Feeding via a PEG tube may be intermittent or continuous. Continuous feeding has been shown to reduce the incidence of diarrhoea (Howell 2002).

3. Bowel sounds should be present before feeding via the PEG is commenced. This is usually 6–12 hours after placement.

4. Avoid adding anything to the feed. If drugs are to be administered via the PEG tube, they must be soluble in water and the tube should be flushed with 50ml of sterile water before and after their administration to prevent blockage.

5. When flushing the PEG tube, care should be taken when attaching the syringe, to avoid damaging the connection. A 20ml (or larger) syringe should be used to flush the tube, as the pressure exerted by smaller syringes is too great. If the PEG tube is not being used for feeding for a period of time, it should be flushed twice a day, to maintain patency.

6. The site should be inspected daily for signs of leakage, swelling, skin irritation or breakdown, soreness or excessive movement of the tube.

7. The administration set must be changed every 24 hours and should be labelled to indicate the date that the change is due.

Bibliography/Suggested reading

Abdulla A, Keast J. Hypodermoclysis as a means of rehydration. *Nursing Times* 1997, **93**(29):54–55.

Arrowsmith H. Nursing management of patients receiving nasogastric feed. *British Journal of Nursing* 1993, **2**(21):1053–1058.

Association of Community Health Councils. Hungry in hospital. *Elderly Care* 1997, **9**(3):22–25.

Bond S (ed). *Eating matters: a resource for improving dietary care in hospitals.* Newcastle upon Tyne: Centre for Health Services Research, 1997.

Burnham P. A guide to nasogastric tube insertion. *Nursing Times* 2000, **98**(8):NT Plus 6–7.

Cotton E, Zinober B, Jessop J. A nutritional assessment tool for older patients. *Professional Nurse* 1996, **11**(9):609–612.

Department of Health. *The essence of care.* London: DoH, 2001.

Donnelly M. The benefits of hypodermoclysis. *Nursing Standard* 1999, **13**(52):44–45.

Holmes S. The incidence of malnutrition in hospitalised patients. *Nursing Times* 1996, **92**(12):43–45.

Howell M. Do nurses know enough about percutaneous endoscopic gastrostomy? *Nursing Times* 2002, **98**(17):40–42.

Jolley S. Managing post-operative nausea and vomiting. *Nursing Standard* 2001, **15**(40):47–55.

Kennedy JF. Enteral feeding for the critically ill patient. *Nursing Standard* 1997, **11**(33):39–43.

Liddle K. Making sense of percutaneous endoscopic gastrostomy. *Nursing Times* 1995, **91**(18):32–33.

Mansfield S. Subcutaneous fluid administration and site maintenance. *Nursing Standard* 1998, **13**(12):56, 59, 60, 62.

McLaren S, Green S. Nutritional screening and assessment. *Professional Nurse Study Supplement* 1998, **13**(6):9–12.

Tate S, Cook H. Post-operative nausea and vomiting 2: management and treatment. *British Journal of Nursing* 1996, **5**(7):1032–1039.

Tate S, Cook H. Post-operative nausea and vomiting 1: physiology and aetiology. *British Journal of Nursing* 1996, **5**(16):962–973.

Walters E. Know how – nutritional assessment. *Nursing Times* 1998, **94**(8):68–69.

Ward J, Rollins H. Screening for malnutrition. *Nursing Standard* 1999, **14**(8):49–53.

Weetch R. Feeding problems in elderly patients. *Nursing Times* 2001, **97**(16):60–61.

Notes

7

Medicines

Principles

In line with legal requirements and local policies, it is part of the nurse's role to ensure that medicines are safely stored. The following principles apply to all situations involving the administration of medicines:

- All medicines, lotions and reagents (except intravenous fluids and drugs for use in emergency situations) must be stored in locked cupboards. Drugs for emergency use (e.g. in cardiac arrest) may be kept with the emergency equipment but must be in a sealed container, which is then replenished and resealed after use.
- All medicines, including emergency drugs and intravenous fluids, must be stored in an environment that meets the manufacturers' recommendations, e.g. temperature.
- Medicine cupboards must be kept locked at all times; drug trolleys must be locked and secured to the wall when not in use, and individual medicines cabinets (sometimes called 'patient's own dispensary') must be locked when not in use.
- Controlled drugs must be kept separate from other medicines, and the key kept separately from other drug keys. A controlled drugs register must also be kept.
- All stock must be rotated so that medicines are used before their expiry date.
- The security of medicines is the responsibility of the nurse in charge. No unauthorised person must be allowed access to the keys (refer to local policy regarding who has authorised access to the keys).

Principles

In some hospitals, patients are given responsibility for taking their own prescribed medicines in preparation for their discharge home. Local policies will differ, but the principles for self-administration of medicines are based upon the availability of individual locked cupboards for storage (usually attached to the patient's locker), a medicines regimen that is not subject to frequent change and individually dispensed medicines from the pharmacy department.

- The nurse's role in self-administration of medicines is to support and educate the patient in the safe administration of their medicines.
- Collaborative working between all members of the healthcare team is imperative if the patient's suitability for self-administration is to be assessed and appropriate education and support provided.
- The nurse must assess the patient's ability to self-administer their medicines prior to entering them into the programme. Most policies for self-administration of medicines include obtaining written consent from the patient before entering them into the programme.
- Many programmes also have varying levels of supervision according to the patient's ability and the level of support and education required. For example, initially the nurse may administer the patient's medicines whilst implementing a planned programme of education. The education programme should include detailed information (both verbal and written) about the medicines, their dosage and times for administration, intended effects and any possible side effects. The written information should include patient information leaflets and also an individualised card indicating the times and dosages for each medicine. During this period the nurse can assess the need for any compliance aids that may be required such as bottle-top openers or large print on labels. The next level of supervision is when patients administer their own medicines under supervision. The final level is when patients administer their own medicines and are given responsibility for the key to their cabinet. It is important that sufficient time is allocated to the programme, so that patients have time to fully understand their medicines prior to discharge home.
- It is thought that planned self-administration programmes whilst patients are in hospital will improve compliance with drug regimens after discharge (Deeks & Byatt 2000).

Drug calculations

It is sometimes necessary to carry out drug calculations in order to administer prescribed medicines correctly, for example when the medicines are not available in the exact dosage that has been prescribed.

Converting from one unit of measurement to another

It is sometimes necessary to convert from one unit of measurement to another in order to be able to administer the correct amount of medicine.

To convert units you need to know the following:

$$
\begin{aligned}
1\,\text{kilogram (kg)} &= 1000 \text{ grams (g)} \\
1 \text{ gram (g)} &= 1000 \text{ milligrams (mg)} \\
1 \text{ milligram} &= 1000 \text{ micrograms (mcg)}
\end{aligned}
$$

To convert grams (g) to milligrams (mg) or milligrams (mg) to micrograms (mcg) you need to multiply by 1000. This is achieved by moving the decimal point three places to the right.

$$\text{e.g. } 6.5\text{mg} \times 1000 = 6500\text{mcg}$$

To convert micrograms (mcg) into milligrams (mg) or milligrams (mg) to grams (g), you need to divide by 1000. This is achieved by moving the decimal point three places to the left.

$$\text{e.g. } 2500\text{mcg} = 2.5\text{mg}$$

Calculating the number of tablets required

In order to calculate the correct number of tablets, use the following formula:

$$\text{number of measures required (i.e. tablets)} = \frac{\text{dose prescribed}}{\text{dose per measure}}$$

Firstly you need to convert the amount required into the same units of measurement as the tablets, then use the formula.

For example, 1g of paracetamol is prescribed. Paracetamol is dispensed in 500mg tablets.

$$1\text{g} = 1000\text{mg}$$

$$\text{Number of tablets} = \frac{1000\text{mg}}{500\text{mg}}$$

$$= 2 \text{ tablets to be given.}$$

Calculating the volume to give

In order to calculate the correct volume, use the following formula:

$$\text{volume to give} = \frac{\text{dose required}}{\text{dose available}} \times \text{volume available}$$

For example 75mg of pethidine is prescribed. Pethidine is dispensed in ampoules containing 100mg in 2ml.

$$\text{volume to give} = \frac{75}{100} \times 2 = 1.5\text{ml}$$

Calculating infusion rates

See IV therapy, Regulation of flow rate (page 66).

The following principles apply to the administration of all medicines, regardless of route.

Preparation

Patient

- Check the location of the patient before dispensing the medication. Do not leave medicines unattended for administration at a later time.
- Check the patient understands the reasons for the medication being administered and any special instructions, e.g. swallow whole or after food, etc.
- Ascertain whether the patient has any drug allergies **PFP1**.
- The patient should be wearing a nameband.

Equipment/Environment

- Medicines to be administered and equipment appropriate to the route of administration.
- Patient's prescription chart.
- Drug reference book, e.g. British National Formulary.

Nurse

- **Medicines may only be administered by a registered nurse PFP2**.
- The nurse must have knowledge of the action, usual dose and side effects of the drugs being administered and knowledge of legislation and local policies relating to the administration of medicines.
- Local policy may require that two nurses check certain medicines before administration.
- Wash and dry hands thoroughly.

Procedure

1. Check the prescription chart has patient's full name and hospital number and read the prescription to ascertain which medicines require administration.
2. Check by which route each medicine is to be given.
3. Check the prescription is dated and is legible and signed by a doctor.
4. Check it is the correct time to administer the medicine and that the patient has not already received it. Check any special observations (e.g. blood pressure) or requirements relating to the medication (e.g. before or after food).
5. Identify the correct medication by checking the medicine container against the prescription chart.
6. Check the expiry date of the medicine.
7. Calculate how much is needed to achieve the prescribed dose (e.g. how many tablets or how much of the ampoule).
8. Repeat steps 2–7 for all medicines due at this time.
9. Check the patient's identity – using the patient's nameband, a photograph or verbally, against the prescription chart, according to local policy.

10. Administer the medicine as prescribed. Medicines must not be left at the bedside unattended. The patient may forget to take them or another patient may take them by mistake.

Post procedure

Patient

- Ensure the patient is comfortable and understands why the medication has been administered.

Equipment/Environment

- Dispose of any packaging and other waste.

Nurse

- Sign/initial the prescription chart according to local policy, to indicate that the medicine has been administered. If the medication cannot be administered for some reason, this must also be documented.
- Monitor the effects of the medication and document in the nursing records. Report any abnormal effects/side effects immediately.

Points for practice

1. If the allergy section of the prescription chart has not been completed, check with the patient and/or the medical notes before administering any medicines. If the patient has no known allergies, this should be indicated in the box, it should not just be left blank.

2. Student nurses may only participate in the administration of medicines under the direct supervision of a registered nurse. A registered nurse must countersign student signatures.

Preparation

Patient

- Ask/assist the patient to assume a position that allows easy swallowing.
- Ensure the patient has plenty of fluid with which to take the medicine.

Equipment/Environment

- Medicines to be administered plus medicine pots, tablet cutter, tissues, jug of water and/or milk if appropriate.
- Prescription chart.

Nurse

- **Only registered nurses may administer medicines** `PFP1`.
- Wash and dry hands thoroughly.

Procedure

1. Check the prescription as described on page 124.
2. Calculate how much liquid or how many tablets or capsules are required to achieve the prescribed dose (see page 122). Do not break tablets unless they are scored across the middle. Break scored tablets with a file, tablet cutter or using a tissue, to avoid handling `PFP2`.
3. Dispense the prescribed amount into a medicine pot. If not in a blister pack, shake the tablets/capsules into the top of the container before transferring to the medicine pot, to avoid handling them (Figure 7.1). Liquid preparations may be drawn up in a syringe for accuracy of measurement.
4. Repeat this procedure for all medicines due at this time.
5. Check the patient's identity – using the patient's nameband or verbally, according to local policy – against the prescription chart.
6. Make sure the patient is in an appropriate position to swallow the medicine and has sufficient fluid.
7. Do not leave medicines unattended at the bedside for later administration.

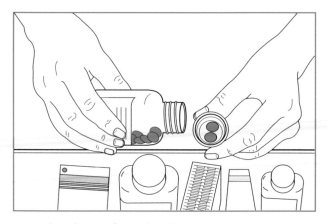

Figure 7.1 Non-touch technique for oral medicines

Post procedure

Patient

- Make sure the patient has taken the medicine as prescribed.

Equipment/Environment

- Dispose of any packaging, disposable medicine pots, etc., in the clinical waste.
- Wash and dry other equipment as necessary and leave ready for use.

Nurse

- Document drugs administered according to local policy.

Points for practice

1. Student nurses may only participate in the administration of medicines under the direct supervision of a registered nurse. A registered nurse must countersign student signatures.

2. Only soluble or dispersible preparations may be dissolved in water. If the patient is unable to swallow whole tablets, the pharmacist should be consulted to identify an alternative preparation, e.g. suspension or elixir. Tablets should not be crushed without first consulting the pharmacist to ascertain whether this is appropriate. Except in exceptional circumstances, medicines for patients who refuse to take them should not be disguised in food (UKCC 2001).

Preparation

Patient

- Explain the procedure, to gain consent and co-operation.
- Check the patient understands the reasons for taking the medication.

Equipment/Environment

- Patient's prescription chart.
- Controlled drugs register.

Nurse

- Ensure knowledge of legislation and local policies relating to the administration of controlled drugs **PFP1,2** .
- Two nurses are usually required, one of whom must be a registered nurse (check local policy).
- Wash and dry hands thoroughly.

Procedure

If local policy stipulates two nurses, they must both be involved in **all** stages of this procedure.

1. Read the prescription chart to ascertain which drugs require administration and by which route.
2. Check that the prescription has the patient's full name and hospital number and is dated, legible and signed by the doctor.
3. Check that it is the correct time to administer the drug and that the patient has not already received it. You may also need to check that the appropriate time has elapsed since the previous dose and any special requirements such as the maximum dosage allowed in 24 hours.
4. Select the appropriate drug from the controlled drugs cupboard, checking that the quantity corresponds with that indicated in the controlled drugs register. Check the expiry date.
5. Remove the drug from its container and check it against the prescription.
6. Check the quantity remaining and replace in the cupboard. Lock the cupboard.
7. Check the amount required, route, time and patient's identity again with the prescription.
8. Select/draw up the correct amount/volume of the drug, performing any calculation as required.
   Any unused portion of an ampoule must be washed down the sink.
9. In the controlled drugs register, record the patient's full name, the dose to be administered (any wastage must also be recorded), the time and the stock number remaining.
10. At the bedside, check that the information on the patient's name band corresponds with that on the prescription. Check again the drug, dose, route and time against the prescription.

11. Administer the drug by the prescribed route. Both nurses must now sign the prescription chart and the controlled drugs register.

Post procedure

Patient

- Ensure the patient is comfortable and is aware of the effects and side effects of the drug.

Equipment/Environment

- Discard all waste appropriately.
- Ensure the controlled drugs register is completed and returned to the appropriate place **PFP3** .

Nurse

- Monitor the effects of the drug and report any side effects immediately.

Points for practice

1. The keys to the controlled drugs cupboard must be kept separately from other keys and must be carried by the nurse in charge of the ward. No unauthorised personnel must have access to these keys.

2. Some drugs are controlled drugs in certain preparations only. For example, intramuscular dihydrocodeine (DF118) is a controlled drug but the oral preparation is not.

3. Controlled-drug registers must not be thrown away when full but must be retained in storage for 5 years. Check local policy for details.

Preparation

Patient

- Explain the procedure, to gain consent and co-operation.
- Ask/assist the patient to choose the site of injection.

Equipment/Environment

- Prescription chart.
- Prescribed drug.
- Cardboard tray or receiver.
- Syringe of appropriate size (0.5–2ml).
- Orange (25G) needle.
- Small clinical wipe/tissue.
- Sharps bin.

Nurse

- **Only registered nurses may administer medicines** PFP1.
- Knowledge of local drug administration policy.
- Wash and dry hands thoroughly.

Procedure

1. Check the drug against the prescription (see page 124) and check the patient's name band.
2. Prepare the syringe as for intramuscular injection (see page 133) PFP2.
3. Select the site of administration (Figure 7.2) PFP3.
4. It is not necessary to clean the skin PFP4. Pinch up the skin using the thumb and first finger of your non-dominant hand and insert the short needle into the subcutaneous tissue at an angle of 80–90° (Figure 7.3).
5. It is not necessary to withdraw the piston as it is unlikely that a blood vessel of any size will be punctured.
6. Inject the solution slowly. On completion, pause briefly before withdrawing the needle as this helps to prevent backtracking.
7. Do not massage the site. If necessary, use the tissue to wipe away any blood.
8. Dispose of the syringe and needle into the sharps bin immediately.

Post procedure

Patient

- Ensure the patient is comfortable.

Equipment/Environment

- Put away all equipment. Some drugs (e.g. insulin) have to be kept in the refrigerator.
- Dispose of waste appropriately.

Nurse

- Sign the prescription to indicate that the drug has been administered.
- Report any abnormalities/complications.

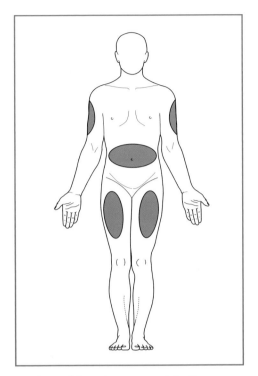

Figure 7.2 Sites commonly used for subcutaneous injection

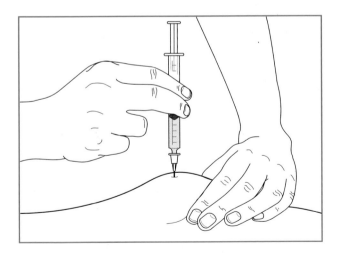

Figure 7.3 Subcutaneous injection technique

Points for practice

1. Only registered nurses may administer medications. Student nurses may only participate in the administration of medicines under the direct supervision of a registered nurse. A registered nurse must countersign student signatures.

2. Some drugs (e.g. heparin) are manufactured in pre-filled syringes. Unlike all other injections, the air in a heparin syringe is not expelled, but is designed to remain in the syringe, by the piston. When the small amount of drug is given, the air fills the needle hub/nozzle of the syringe and needle. This prevents the drug tracking back to the surface as the needle is withdrawn and causing skin irritation.

3. Patients receiving regular subcutaneous injections (e.g. insulin) will wish to rotate the injection site. Possible sites are the upper arms, the anterior aspect of the thighs, and the abdomen (see Figure 7.2). Heparin is usually given into the subcutaneous tissue of the abdominal wall.

4. The skin is not cleaned because, with repeated use, alcohol causes the skin to harden and many patients will be having subcutaneous injections over a long period of time, possibly for the rest of their life.

Preparation

Patient

- Explain the procedure, to gain consent and co-operation.
- Check the patient's understanding of the reason for the injection.

Equipment/Environment

- Prescription chart.
- Prescribed medicine and diluent if required.
- Cardboard tray or receiver.
- Sterile syringe of appropriate size (2–5ml).
- Sterile needle – usually green (21G) for adult patients **PFP1**.
- Alcohol-impregnated swab.
- Small clinical wipe/tissue.
- Sharps bin.

Nurse

- **Only registered nurses may administer medicines.** A second nurse may be required depending on the local drug administration policy **PFP2**.
- Wash and dry hands thoroughly.
- Gloves may be required depending on the type of drug being given (e.g. antibiotics).

Procedure

1. Check the medicine and any diluent against the prescription chart (see checking procedure, page 124).
2. Open the syringe packaging at the plunger end and remove the syringe. Check that the plunger will move freely inside the barrel.
3. Taking care not to touch the nozzle end, hold the syringe in one hand and open the needle packaging at the hilt (coloured) end. Attach the needle firmly to the syringe and loosen, but do not remove, the cover. Place in the tray/receiver.
4. If a glass ampoule of liquid is being used, ensure that all the contents are in the bottom of the ampoule, then break off the top, using a clinical wipe/tissue or syringe wrapper to protect your fingers. If a plastic ampoule is being used, break off the top, taking care not to touch the top of the ampoule with your fingers.
5. Pick up the syringe and needle and allow the needle cover to slide off into the tray or receiver.
6. Carefully insert the needle through the neck of the ampoule and into the solution, taking care not to allow it to scrape against the bottom of the ampoule, as this blunts the needle.
7. Draw back on the plunger, using your thumb and middle finger on the plunger with your first finger against the flange of the syringe, until the required amount is in the syringe.
8. If the medicine is in powder form, draw up the diluent, clean the rubber stopper of the ampoule/vial with an alcohol-impregnated swab and allow

it to dry. Inject a small amount of diluent (usually 1.5–2ml) into the ampoule/vial. Mix thoroughly by gently agitating or rolling the ampoule/vial until all the powder has dissolved **PFP3**.

9. Holding the ampoule/vial upside down at eye level, pull back the plunger to draw the liquid into the syringe. Make sure that the needle remains below the surface of the liquid to prevent air being drawn into the syringe (Figure 7.4).

10. Replace the ampoule in tray/receiver. Taking care not to touch the needle with your hand, carefully resheathe the needle using the non-touch method (Figure 7.5) **PFP4**.

11. Hold the syringe upright at eye level and encourage any air to rise to the top of the syringe. Gently tap the barrel of the syringe if necessary to make air bubbles rise to the top. Expel the air by gently pressing the plunger until droplets of liquid are seen at the top of the needle (Figure 7.6).

12. Take the tray/receiver containing the syringe, ampoule and alcohol-impregnated swab plus the sharps bin to the patient. Check the medicine and prescription again and the patient's nameband.

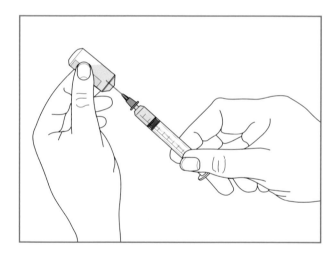

Figure 7.4 Drawing up the injection

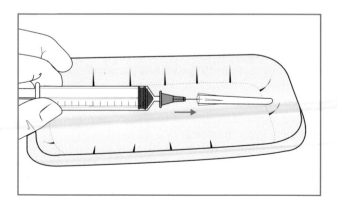

Figure 7.5 Safe re-sheathing technique

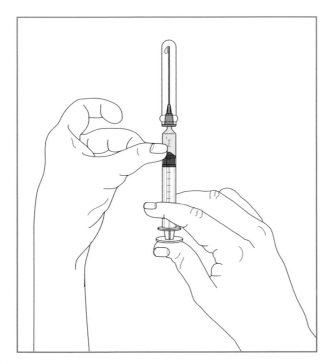

Figure 7.6 Expelling the air

13. Ensure privacy. Select the site and ask/assist the patient to adopt a suitable position (Figure 7.7) **PFP5**.
14. Clean the skin with the alcohol-impregnated swab and allow to dry **PFP6**.
15. Stretch the skin slightly with your non-dominant hand.
16. Holding the syringe like a dart in your dominant hand, warn the patient, then insert the needle swiftly and firmly at an angle of 90° to the skin, leaving about 1cm of the needle showing (Figure 7.8).
17. With the ulnar border of your hand against the skin, hold the coloured part of the needle to prevent movement.
18. Withdraw the plunger slightly to check the needle has not inadvertently entered a blood vessel **PFP7**.
19. Depress the plunger steadily, not too quickly, until the syringe is empty.
20. Quickly and smoothly withdraw the needle from the skin and press firmly on the site with the swab or a tissue until any bleeding stops.
21. Do not resheathe the needle. Discard it, still attached to the syringe, into the sharps bin.

Post procedure

Patient

- Assist the patient into a comfortable position and replace clothing as necessary.
- Intramuscular medicines given will usually take effect within 20 minutes. Check for the desired effect and for side effects, especially if an analgesic or anti-emetic.

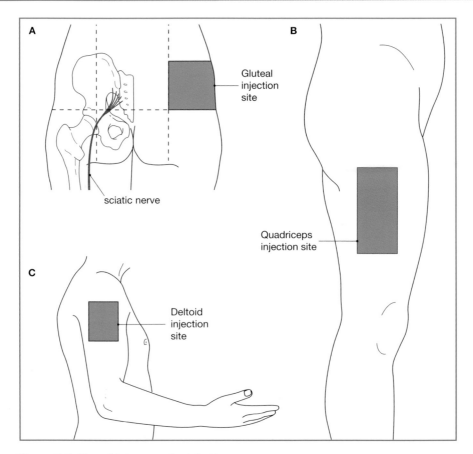

Figure 7.7 Sites of intramuscular injection

Equipment/Environment

• Discard all used equipment appropriately.

Nurse

• Wash hands.
• Sign/initial the prescription chart to indicate that the medicine has been given.

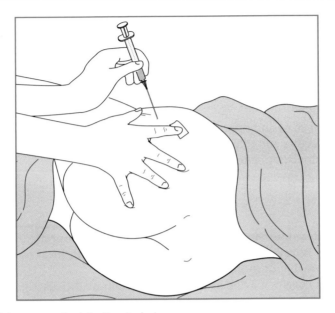

Figure 7.8 Intramuscular injection technique

Points for practice

1. If the patient is very thin or cachexic, the same gauge needle is used but it is not inserted so deeply.

2. Each Trust will have its own drug administration policy, which will indicate whether two nurses are required to check certain drugs. It will also indicate the role of the student nurse in drug administration.

3. When mixing the medicine, keep the needle inside the ampoule so that it remains sterile. If there is pressure within the vial, you may need to keep your thumb on the plunger.

4. Resheathing the needle before administration to the patient is quite safe and ensures that droplets of the drug are not inhaled or sprayed onto the skin as air is expelled from the syringe.

5. The most common sites for intramuscular injection are the gluteus maximus and the lateral aspects of the vastus lateralis (one of the quadriceps). Smaller intramuscular injections, such as vaccinations, are usually given into the deltoid area (see Figure 7.7).

6. Some local policies no longer recommend skin cleansing prior to IM injection because they regard it as unnecessary if the skin is clean (Little 2000).

7. If blood appears in the syringe at step 18, stop, withdraw the needle and start the procedure again with a new syringe and drug. This happens only very rarely.

Preparation

Patient

- Explain the procedure, to gain consent and co-operation.
- The patient should be resting in a chair or in bed.

Equipment/Environment

- Prescription chart and prescribed medicines.
- Syringes, needles and diluents as appropriate.
- 0.9% Sodium chloride to flush the cannula **PFP1**.
- Alcohol-impregnated swab.
- Sharps bin.

Nurse

- **Only registered nurses who have undergone the appropriate training may administer intravenous medicines in accordance with local policies** **PFP2**.
- Wash and dry hands thoroughly.
- Gloves and goggles may be necessary with certain medicines, e.g. cytotoxic drugs.

Procedure

1. Check the medicine as described on page 124. Whether you need to check these with another nurse will depend on the local intravenous drug administration policy **PFP2**.
2. Prepare the medicine for administration, checking the expiry date of all medicines and any diluents used. Prepare 10ml of 0.9% sodium chloride flush (more if several medicines are to be administered) **PFP1**.
3. At the bedside, check the medicine and the patient's name band against the prescription again.
4. Adopt a comfortable posture (sitting is probably best) in a position that allows easy access to the cannula. Face the patient so that any adverse reaction may be observed, and if the patient is undergoing cardiac monitoring, this should also be in view.
5. Check the cannula site for signs of infection, phlebitis or discomfort/pain. If the site is bandaged, the bandage must be removed to allow inspection of the site. If there is an infusion running, the intravenous bolus may be administered via the small injection port that is situated approximately 10 cm from the end of the administration set. If this is used, the infusion must be stopped while the bolus is administered as described below, and then recommenced at the prescribed rate **PFP3**.
6. Thoroughly disinfect the rubber membrane of the injection port or injectable cap/bung according to local policy (Figure 7.9) **PFP4**.
7. Before administering the medicine, administer a small amount (1–2ml) of the 0.9% sodium chloride flush to confirm the patency of the cannula. If resistance is felt, do not continue as this may dislodge a clot at the end of the cannula **PFP5**.

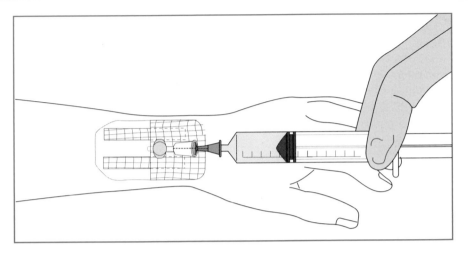

Figure 7.9 Intravenous drug administration

8. Slowly administer the medicine according to the prescription, the manufacturer's instructions, and/or local policies and procedures, using a small (25G) needle through the injectable rubber cap or port **PFP6** .
9. Administer the remaining flush or, if a number of medicines are being given, flush between each one to prevent mixing in the cannula.

Post procedure

Patient

• Ensure the patient is comfortable.
• Advise the patient to report any side effects.

Equipment/Environment

• Dispose of needles, glass ampoules, etc., immediately into a sharps bin.

Nurse

• Document the drug administration according to local policies and procedures.

Points for practice

1. 0.9% Sodium chloride is used for flushing purposes except in a few instances when the drug being administered is incompatible with sodium chloride. In these cases (e.g. amphotericin), 5% glucose should be used instead. In many NHS Trusts, the 0.9% sodium chloride or 5% glucose flush may be administered without prescription.

2. Although single-nurse administration is common for other routes of administration, some local policies require two nurses to administer intravenous drugs. It is vital that both nurses check thoroughly – you should never rely on the other nurse to check that it is correct.

3. If the infusion is prescribed to run at a very slow rate (e.g. dobutamine) it is better to use a separate cannula for bolus IV medications. If this is not possible, administer the flush and the bolus at a slower rate than the infusion to ensure that the infusion is not given faster than the prescribed rate.

4. Although some cannulae have an integral injection port, this should not be used for drug administration as it is difficult to keep the port clean and provides a reservoir for bacterial contamination.

5. If the patient complains of pain at the site, this may be due to infiltration or extravasation. If a small amount of flush solution is administered before the medicine to test patency, it will only be 0.9% sodium chloride rather than some potentially more damaging substance that is administered into the surrounding tissues.

6. There are a number of 'needle-free' injection caps available. These allow the syringe to be fitted directly into the injection cap without the need for a needle, thus reducing the risk of a needle-stick injury.

Preparation

Patient

- Explain the procedure, to gain consent and co-operation.
- Ask the patient to lie down or sit in a chair where they will be able to hyper-extend their neck. A pillow under the shoulders is beneficial.

Equipment/Environment

- Prescription chart.
- Nose drops as prescribed.
- Clean tissues.

Nurse

- **Only registered nurses may administer medicines** PFP1,2
- Wash and dry hands thoroughly.

Procedure

1. Check the drops against the prescription chart (see page 124), noting whether the drops are to be instilled into one or both nostrils.
2. Ask the patient to hyperextend their neck.
3. Remove the cap from the nose drops container.
4. Using the dropper, administer the correct number of drops into each nostril, taking care not to touch the nose with the dropper PFP3.
5. Ask the patient to remain in this position for at least 2 minutes to allow absorption of the medication.
6. Wipe away any excess medication with a tissue.

Post procedure

Patient

- Ensure the patient is comfortable PFP4.
- Ask the patient to refrain from blowing their nose for 20 minutes following the procedure if possible.

Equipment/Environment

- Discard any used tissues into the clinical waste.
- Return the nose drops to the correct storage area.

Nurse

- Wash and dry hands thoroughly.
- Record administration on the prescription chart.
- Evaluate the effect of the nose drops and document in the nursing records if appropriate.
- Report any abnormalities.

Points for practice

1. Only registered nurses may administer medications. Student nurses may only participate in the administration of nose drops under the direct supervision of a registered nurse. A registered nurse must countersign student signatures.

2. Patients may be able to administer nose drops themselves. Nurses should ensure that they are using the correct procedure (see self-administration of medicines, page 121)

3. It may be necessary to clean the nasal passages before administration of nose drops. This can be achieved by asking the patient to blow their nose or by using gauze moistened with 0.9% sodium chloride or water.

4. Nose drops may run into the back of the throat, causing the patient to experience an unusual taste.

Preparation

Patient

- Explain the procedure, to gain consent and co-operation.
- Explain the action of the ear drops and the expected outcome.
- Ask the patient to sit upright with their head tilted slightly away from the affected ear or to lie on their side with the affected ear uppermost.

Equipment/Environment

- Prescription chart
- Ear drops as prescribed **PFP1**.
- Clean tissues.

Nurse

- **Only registered nurses may administer medicines** **PFP2**.
- Wash and dry hands thoroughly.

Procedure

1. Check the ear drops against the prescription chart, noting which ear is to have the drops instilled (see page 124).
2. Remove the cap from the ear drops container.
3. Gently pull the pinna of the ear upwards and backwards.
4. Squeeze the bottle or dropper to dispense the prescribed number of drops into the ear taking care not to touch the skin with the dropper.
5. Release the pinna.
6. Replace the cap.
7. Instruct the patient to remain in this position for 1–2 minutes to allow the drops to reach the eardrum.
8. When the patient is sitting upright, use the tissue to wipe away any excess fluid from the outer ear.
9. If prescribed, repeat the process in the other ear after 5–10 minutes **PFP3**.

Post procedure

Patient

- Ensure the patient is comfortable.

Equipment/Environment

- Store the eardrops in the appropriate place.
- Dispose of clinical waste appropriately.

Nurse

- Wash and dry hands thoroughly.
- Record administration on the prescription chart.
- Evaluate the effect of the eardrops and document in the nursing records if appropriate.
- Report any abnormalities.

Points for practice

1. If both ears require drops, there may be a separate bottle for each ear.

2. Only registered nurses may administer medications. Student nurses may only participate in the administration of ear drops under the direct supervision of a registered nurse. A registered nurse must countersign student signatures.

3. Patients may be able to administer ear drops themselves. Nurses should ensure that they are using the correct procedure (see self-administration of medicines, page 121).

Preparation

Patient

- Explain the procedure, to gain consent and co-operation.
- Instruct the patient to tilt their head backwards and look up.
- Explain that vision may be blurred for a short while after administration of the drops/ointment.

Equipment/Environment

- Prescription chart.
- Eye drops or ointment as prescribed **PFP1,2**.
- Clean tissues.

Nurse

- **Only registered nurses may administer medicines PFP3**.
- Wash and dry hands thoroughly.

Procedure

1. Check the eye drops against the prescription, noting which eye is to have the drops/ointment instilled (see page 124).
2. Remove the cap from the drops/ointment container.
3. Using your forefinger, gently pull the lower lid downwards to form a small pocket for the drops/ointment.
4. Hold the tissue beneath the eye.
5. Hold the dispenser between your thumb and forefinger about 2–3cm from the patient's eye.
6. Eye-drops – squeeze one drop into the eye and ask the patient to blink before the next drop. Repeat until the prescribed number of drops has been administered (Figure 7.10a).
   Eye ointment – squeeze the tube gently until a small amount (about 1–2cm) of ointment forms a 'ribbon'. Apply the ribbon inside the lid margin, from the inner to outer aspect of the eye (Figure 7.10B). Do not touch any part of the eye with the tube.
7. Ask the patient to close (but not squeeze) their eyes for a few seconds to disperse the medication.
8. Wipe away any excess medication that runs down the cheek with a clean tissue.
9. Replace the cap.
10. If more than one medication is required, repeat the process after 2–3 minutes **PFP4**.

Post procedure

Patient

- Ensure the patient is comfortable and that vision has returned to normal.

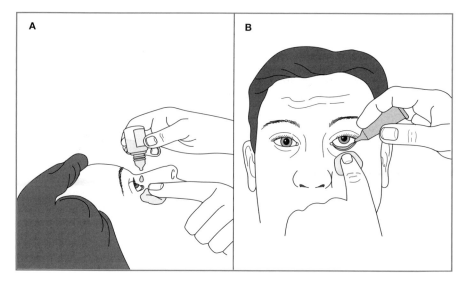

Figure 7.10 A = Administration of eye drops
B = Administration of eye ointment

Equipment/Environment

- Store the eye drops/ointment in the appropriate place (eye drops may be kept in the refrigerator once opened).
- Discard tissues into clinical waste.

Nurse

- Wash and dry hands thoroughly.
- Record administration on the prescription chart.
- Evaluate the effect of the eye drops/ointment and document in the nursing records if appropriate.
- Report any abnormalities.

Points for practice

1. If both eye drops and eye ointment are to be administered, administer the eye drops first as the grease base of the ointment can inhibit the absorption of drops.

2. If both eyes are being treated, there may be a separate bottle/tube for each eye.

3. Only registered nurses may administer medications. Student nurses may only participate in the administration of eye drops/ointment under the direct supervision of a registered nurse. A registered nurse must countersign student signatures.

4. Patients may be able to administer eye drops themselves. Nurses should ensure that they are using the correct procedure (see self-administration of medicines, page 121).

Preparation

Patient

- Explain the procedure, to gain co-operation and consent.
- If possible patients should apply the cream or ointment themselves. The nurse should ensure they are applying it correctly.

Equipment/Environment

- Ensure the screens are pulled round to promote dignity and comfort.
- Prescription chart.
- Cream, ointment, lotion or topical patch as prescribed.
- Gloves or sterile gauze to apply cream/lotion/ointment.

Nurse

- **Only registered nurses may administer medicines** PFP1 .
- Wash and dry hands thoroughly.
- Put on gloves.

Procedure

1. Check the medicine against the prescription chart (see page 124 for procedure).
2. Locate the appropriate part of the body. If a topical patch is used, remove backing and apply the patch to clean, dry skin. If cream, ointment or lotion, rub in with a piece of sterile gauze, wearing gloves to avoid absorption of the active ingredients PFP2 .

Post procedure

Patient

- Ensure the patient is comfortable.

Equipment/Environment

- Discard gloves and gauze in clinical waste.

Nurse

- Wash and dry hands thoroughly.
- Document that medicine has been administered and note condition of skin.

Points for practice

1. Only registered nurses may administer medications. Student nurses may only participate in the administration of topical applications under the direct supervision of a registered nurse. A registered nurse must countersign student signatures.

2. If the medicine comes in the form of a topical patch, the site of application should be varied according to the manufacturer's instructions, i.e. the same site should not be used on consecutive applications and the patch may need to be removed after a certain time period.

Preparation

Patient

- Explain the procedure, to gain co-operation and consent.
- Wherever possible the woman should be assisted as necessary to administer the cream or pessary herself. If this is not possible, ask/assist her to lie on her back with her knees up and legs apart.

Equipment/Environment

- Ensure the screens are pulled round to promote dignity and comfort.
- Prescription chart.
- Cream or pessary as prescribed.
- Vaginal applicator.
- Gauze swabs or tissues.
- Protective pad or panty liner.

Nurse

- **Only registered nurses may administer medicines** `PFP1`.
- Wash and dry hands thoroughly.
- Put on gloves and apron.

Procedure

1. Check the medicine against the prescription chart (see page 124 for procedure).
2. Remove the pessary from the packaging and insert into the applicator. If using a vaginal cream, this is usually pre-loaded in the applicator.
3. Locate the vagina and gently insert the applicator as far as is comfortable.
4. Press the plunger to release the pessary or cream high in the vagina (Figure 7.11).
5. Remove the applicator and wipe away any traces of cream.

Post procedure

Patient

- Ensure patient is comfortable and has a panty liner or pad to protect their underwear.
- Ask patient to remain recumbent for as long as possible `PFP2`.

Equipment/Environment

- Discard vaginal applicator in clinical waste.

Nurse

- Remove gloves and apron.
- Wash and dry hands thoroughly.
- Document that medicine has been administered.

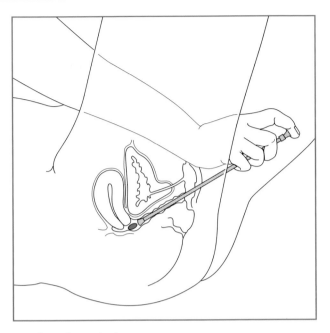

Figure 7.11 Insertion of a vaginal pessary

Points for practice

1. Only registered nurses may administer medications. Student nurses may only participate in the administration of vaginal preparations under the direct supervision of a registered nurse. A registered nurse must countersign student signatures.

2. Vaginal preparations are best administered last thing at night, when the patient will be recumbent for several hours, to allow absorption of the medication.

Preparation

Patient

- Explain the procedure, to gain consent and co-operation.
- Draw the screens and ensure warmth and privacy.
- Ask/assist patient to remove clothing below the waist, and lie in the left lateral position.
- Place an absorbent pad under the buttocks.

Equipment/Environment

- Prescription chart.
- Suppositories as prescribed **PFP2,1**.
- Cardboard tray or receiver.
- Lubricant.
- Gauze swabs or tissues.

Nurse

- **Only registered nurses may administer medicines** **PFP2**.
- Wash and dry hands thoroughly.
- Put on apron and gloves.

Procedure

1. Remove packaging around suppository.
2. Squeeze some lubricant onto a piece of gauze and lubricate the suppository.
3. Warn the patient that he/she will feel suppository being inserted into the rectum.
4. Ask patient to relax; encouraging deep breathing may help.
5. With your left hand, part the buttocks and inspect the anal area so as to avoid skin tags, haemorrhoids, etc. **PFP3**.
6. Gently insert the suppository into the anal canal blunt end first **PFP4**, using the index finger of your right hand (Figure 7.12).

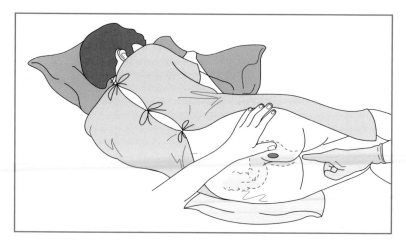

Figure 7.12 Administration of suppositories

7. Repeat the process if more than one suppository is required.
8. Wipe away excess traces of lubricant from the anal area and remove gloves.
9. If it is an evacuant suppository (e.g. glycerine or bisacodyl) leave the patient in a comfortable position with a call bell at hand. To be effective, the suppositories should remain in position for at least 15 minutes and patients should be discouraged from opening their bowels before this time.
10. If the suppository is for drug administration (e.g. paracetamol) the bowel should be opened prior to administration. This suppository is designed to be absorbed through the rectal wall and so the patient should be discouraged from opening their bowels for at least 30 minutes.

Post procedure

Patient

- If the patient is unable to use the lavatory, assist them to use a bedpan/commode as necessary.
- Offer a bowl of water to wash hands.

Equipment/Environment

- Dispose of waste and equipment appropriately.

Nurse

- Remove apron and wash hands.
- Note bowel action following the suppository and document/report result.

Points for practice

1. If the suppository is for drug administration, this must be prescribed and checked as described on page 124.

2. Only registered nurses may administer medications. Student nurses may only participate in the administration of suppositories under the direct supervision of a registered nurse. A registered nurse must countersign student signatures.

3. It is necessary for the patient to be in the left lateral position because of the position of the rectum. This means that for effective insertion, even left-handed nurses must use their right hand to insert the suppository.

4. There is evidence to suggest that if the suppository is inserted blunt end first, insertion and retention of the suppository is easier (Moppett 2000).

Preparation

Patient

- Explain the procedure, to gain co-operation and consent.
- Patients should use inhalers themselves, the nurse's role is to ensure they utilise the correct technique.

Equipment/Environment

- Metered dose inhaler and any adjuncts **PFP1** .
- Prescription chart.

Nurse

- **Only registered nurses may administer medicines** **PFP2** .
- Hands should be clean.

Procedure

1. Check the inhaler against the prescription chart (see page 124 for procedure).
2. Instruct patient to remove cap and shake inhaler. They should then breathe out and make a seal around the mouthpiece (Figure 7.13). As they start to inhale, they should press the canister and hold their breath for a minimum of 10 seconds.

Post procedure

Patient

- Ensure the patient is comfortable.

Equipment/Environment

- Replace the cap and place the inhaler in patient's medicine cupboard.

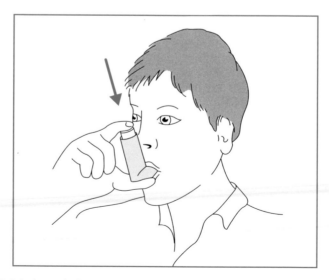

Figure 7.13 Inhaler technique

Nurse

• Document that medicine has been administered.

Points for practice

1. Adjuncts such as a volumatic spacer device can be used for patients who are very breathless or find it difficult to co-ordinate pressing the canister and breathing. Specialist respiratory nurses will be able to advise on other suitable inhaler devices should the patient have difficulty using a metered dose inhaler.

2. Only registered nurses may administer medications. Student nurses may only participate in the administration of inhaled medications under the direct supervision of a registered nurse. A registered nurse must countersign student signatures.

Some patients are unable to take nourishment and medicines orally. If they have a nasogastric tube, medicines may be administered via this route. It is imperative that the pharmacist is consulted to determine whether tablets may be crushed and mixed with water or whether alternative solutions such as suspensions and elixirs are available (Naysmith & Nicholson 1998). You should also consider whether any interaction with the feed may occur and the possibility of blockage of the tube (Cannaby et al 2002). See nasogastric feeding (page 110) for technique.

Bibliography/Suggested reading

Bryson E. Drug administration via a nasogastric tube. *Nursing Times* 2001, 97(16):51.

Campbell J. Injections: techniques and procedures. *Professional Nurse* 1995, 10(7):455–458.

Cannaby AM, Evans L. Freeman A. Nursing care of patients with nasogastric feeding tubes. *British Journal of Nursing* 2002, 11:366–372.

Clarke A. The nursing management of intravenous drug therapy. *British Journal of Nursing* 1997, 6(4): 201–206.

Conaghan P. Subcutaneous heparin injections – bruising. *Surgical Nurse* 1993, 6(2):25–27.

Davis S. Self-administration of medicines. *Nursing Standard* 1991, 5(15):29–31.

Deeks PA, Byatt K. Are patients who self-administer their medicines in hospital more satisfied with their care? *Journal of Advanced Nursing* 2000, 13(2):395–400.

Dickerson RJ. Ten tips for easing the pain of intramuscular injections. *Nursing* 1992, 22(8):55.

Kelly J. Topical ophthalmic drug administration: a practical guide. *British Journal of Nursing* 1994, 4(10):518–520.

Little K. Skin preparation for intramuscular injections. *Nursing Times* 2000, 96(46):NTPlus: 6, 8.

Marsden J. Correct administration of topical eye treatment. *Nursing Standard* 2003, 17(30):42–44.

McConnell EA. Administering subcutaneous heparin. *Nursing* 1990, 20(12):24.

Misuse of Drugs Act. London: HMSO; 1971.

Misuse of Drugs Regulations. London: HMSO; 1985.

Moppett, S. Which way is up for a suppository? *Nursing Times* 2000, 96(19):NTPlus: 12–13.

Naysmith M R, Hicholson J. Nasogastric drug administration. *Professional Nurse* 1998, 13(7):424–427.

Nursing & Midwifery Council. *Guidelines for the administration of medicines.* London, NMC; 2002. Available at nmc-uk.org.uk

Pope BB. How to administer subcutaneous and intramuscular injections: use these techniques to make sure the drug or vaccine gets where it belongs. *Nursing* 2002, 32(1):50–51.

Rodger MA, King L. Drawing up and administering intramuscular injections: a review of the literature. *Journal of Advanced Nursing* 2000, 31(3):574–582.

UKCC. *Position statement on the covert administration of medicines: disguising medicine in food and drink.* London: UKCC; 2001.

Webb R. Treating vaginal infections. *Community Nurse* 1995, 1(9):28.

Williams A. How to avoid mistakes in medicine administration. *Nursing Times* 1996, 92(13):40–42.

Notes

8

Elimination

Principles

Normal faeces (also known as a 'stool') is brown, soft and formed and has an odour but should not be offensive smelling. When observing faeces, the following should be noted and any abnormality reported.

- Amount – particularly if diarrhoea, as patients may lose a lot of fluid this way.
- Frequency – the 'normal' frequency will vary from patient to patient.
- Consistency – the normal consistency is soft and formed. The following should be noted: hard faeces (constipation); liquid (diarrhoea); mucus evident (ulcerative colitis or Crohn's disease); fatty, offensive smelling and floats (steatorrhoea, seen in biliary disease); whether parasites are present.
- Colour – a pale, putty colour suggests the absence of bile pigments. The presence of bright-red blood may indicate bleeding from haemorrhoids or rectal bleeding. If the stool appears black and tarry in consistency (melaena), this indicates digested blood from the stomach or small intestine. If the stool is black and hard in consistency, this may be the result of iron medication.
- Pain/discomfort associated with a bowel action.
- Flatus – the presence of this indicates gut motility and is an important observation following abdominal surgery.

Preparation

Patient

- Explain the procedure, to gain consent and co-operation.

Equipment/Environment

- Sterile stool specimen container.
- Specimen bag.
- Completed pathology request form, e.g. microbiology.

Nurse

- Put on apron and gloves.

Procedure

1. Ask/assist the patient to use a bedpan or commode (see pages 162–166).
2. In the sluice, open the sterile specimen container and remove the spatula (usually attached to the lid of the container) **PFP1**.
3. Use the spatula to remove a small quantity of faeces from the bedpan. Place the faeces and the spatula in the container and secure the lid.
4. Complete the patient's details on the label of the container. If a series of specimens is being collected, ensure the correct sequence is identified.
5. Place the specimen container in the specimen bag, seal it and insert the pathology request form into the pocket **PFP2,3**.

Post procedure

Patient

- Ensure the patient is comfortable.

Equipment/Environment

- Dispose of excreta and place bedpan in the washer or disposal system as appropriate.
- Clean the commode, if used, according to local policy.
- Place specimen in refrigerator to await transport to the laboratory.

Nurse

- Remove gloves and apron and wash hands.
- Document that specimen has been collected.

Points for practice

1. If no spatula is provided, use a disposable wooden tongue depressor.

2. For certain investigations, more than one specimen will be required (e.g. three specimens are required for occult blood).

3. Occasionally, testing for occult blood is done on the ward. The manufacturer's instructions should be followed.

Preparation

Patient

- Explain the procedure, to gain consent and co-operation.
- Draw screens to ensure privacy.
- Ask/assist the patient to remove clothing below the waist and lie in the left lateral position.
- Cover the patient with a blanket.
- Place an absorbent pad under the buttocks.

Equipment/Environment

- Prescription chart **PFP1**.
- Enema as prescribed (Figure 8.1).
- Cardboard tray/receiver.
- Gauze swabs/tissues.
- Lubricant.
- Bedpan or commode, plus toilet paper.

Nurse

- Wash and dry hands thoroughly.
- Put on apron and gloves.

Procedure

1. Check the anal area for soreness, haemorrhoids or skin tags.
2. Remove the cap and lubricate the end of the nozzle.
3. Ask the patient to relax and take deep breaths.

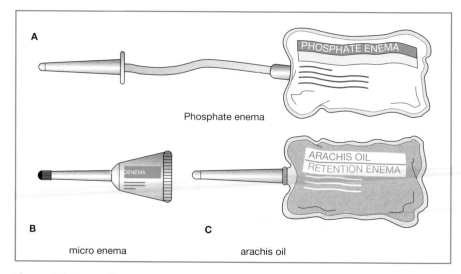

Figure 8.1 Types of enema

4. Part the buttocks with the left hand. With the right hand, hold the nozzle of the enema and *gently* insert it through the anus and into the anal canal PFP2,3 .

5. Squeeze the bag/pack until all the contents have been deposited – the bag/pack may be rolled (like a tube of toothpaste) to expel the last of the contents.

6. While still squeezing and keeping the bag rolled, gently withdraw the nozzle PFP4 .

7. Wipe away any residual lubricant and leave the patient dry. Cover the patient.

8. If it is an evacuant enema, ask the patient to hold the enema for as long as possible but the effect is likely to be rapid. Assist the patient onto the bed-pan or commode as necessary.

If it is a retention enema (drug administration), the patient should be instructed to stay in the left lateral position for at least 30 minutes to aid retention and absorption of the fluid. Raising the foot of the bed may also help.

Post procedure

Patient

- The patient may feel faint and/or nauseous.
- Offer a bowl of water to wash hands after using the bedpan/commode.

Equipment/Environment

- Dispose of clinical waste appropriately.

Nurse

- Remove gloves and apron.
- Wash hands.
- Document/report the result of the enema.

Points for practice

1. If the enema is for drug administration, this must be prescribed and checked as described on page 124.

2. Some enemas may need to be warmed before administration. Do this by placing in warm water.

3. It is necessary for the patient to be in the left lateral position because of the position of the rectum. This means that for effective administration, even left-handed nurses must use their right hand to insert the nozzle of the enema.

4. Keeping the bag rolled while removing the nozzle on completion of the enema, prevents fluid running back into the bag.

Preparation

Patient

- Assess the patient to determine the type of bedpan required – standard or slipper type **PFP1** .
- Ensure privacy and dignity are maintained throughout.

Equipment/Environment

- Clear the bed area.
- Bedpan and cover.
- Toilet paper.

Nurse

- An apron should be worn.
- Gloves should be worn when handling the bedpan and assisting with toileting.
- Some patients may require two nurses for this procedure.

Procedure

1. Take the covered bedpan and toilet paper to the bedside.
2. Ensure the screens are completely drawn.
3. Ask/assist the patient to raise their buttocks and place the bedpan underneath the patient's pelvis – wide rim of bedpan under the buttocks, and narrow area between legs (Figure 8.2).
4. If using a slipper bedpan (Figure 8.3), assist the patient to roll to one side and slip the bedpan underneath from the side; talcum powder applied to the bedpan will assist this process if the patient is sweating. The handle end should be positioned towards the legs.

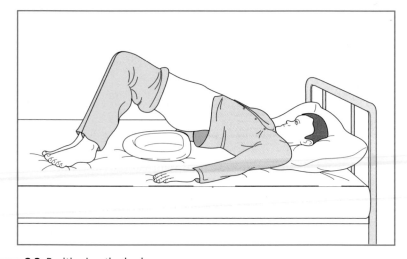

Figure 8.2 Positioning the bedpan

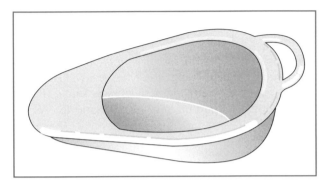

Figure 8.3 The slipper bedpan

5. For female patients, make sure that the legs are slightly apart, otherwise urine may trickle down the legs onto the sheet. For male patients, ensure that the penis is positioned over the bedpan.
6. Preserve the patient's privacy and dignity by covering the patient with the bedclothes.
7. Ensure the call bell is within easy reach and leave the patient but remain within earshot.
8. When the patient has finished, provide assistance with cleansing as necessary and remove the bedpan.
9. Washing with soap and water will be required if the patient has had a bowel action.

Post procedure

Patient

- Ensure patient comfort – straighten the bottom sheet, rearrange pillows, bedclothes, etc., as necessary.
- Offer the patient a bowl of water to wash hands.

Equipment/Environment

- Measure urine if necessary.
- Dispose of excreta safely and place the bedpan in the washer or disposal system as appropriate.
- Return the bedside table and belongings to within easy reach of patient.

Nurse

- Remove gloves and apron and wash hands.
- Record urine output or bowel action if appropriate.

Points for practice

1. The slipper bedpan is used for patients who are unable to sit on a standard bedpan. Its wedge shape makes it easier to insert and more comfortable to use. It is inserted with the handle under the patient's legs and the smooth, flat part underneath the buttocks.

Preparation

Patient

- Assess the level of assistance needed to use the commode.

Equipment/Environment

- Clear the bed area and draw the screens to ensure privacy.
- Commode containing clean bedpan.
- Toilet paper.

Nurse

- An apron should be worn.
- Gloves should be worn when assisting with toileting and removing the commode.

Procedure

1. Take the commode (with seat in place, covering bedpan) and toilet paper to the bedside **PFP1**.
2. Position the commode so that the patient has sufficient room to get out of bed without banging their legs and apply the brakes.
3. Ensure the screens are completely drawn.
4. Check the bed brakes are on.
5. Adjust the bed height to suit the patient.
6. Assist the patient to a sitting position on the edge of the bed.
7. Offer slippers and dressing gown.
8. Assist the patient as necessary to transfer to the commode.
9. If the patient is frail, reposition the commode so that the patient is close to and facing the bed, then apply the brakes and place a pillow at the edge of the bed for the patient to lean on.
10. Provide privacy by leaving, but ensure the patient has access to a call bell and remain within earshot.
11. When the patient has finished, assist with cleaning/washing as necessary.

Post procedure

Patient

- Assist the patient back to bed and offer a hand wash.
- Rearrange pillows, bedclothes, bedside table, etc., as necessary.

Equipment/Environment

- Measure urine if required.
- Dispose of excreta safely and place the bedpan in the washer or disposal system as appropriate.
- Clean the commode according to local policy **PFP2**.

Nurse

- Remove gloves and apron and wash hands.
- Record urine output or bowel action if appropriate.

Points for practice

1. Placing the toilet roll in a small bowl or receiver will prevent it rolling off the commode when being wheeled to the bedside.

2. Local policy for cleaning the commode may vary but cleaning with hot soapy water followed by thorough drying is usually sufficient.

Preparation

Patient

- Explain the procedure, to gain consent and co-operation.
- Assess the patient's level of mobility and ability to assist with the procedure.

Equipment/Environment

- Urinal and cover.
- Provide privacy.

Nurse

- Hands should be clean and an apron and gloves should be worn.

Procedure

1. Ask/assist the patient to adopt an appropriate position. Standing is best if this is possible **PFP1**.
2. If necessary, assist the patient to hold the urinal and position the penis inside.
3. When the patient has finished urinating, remove the urinal and implement the patient's normal cleansing routine.

Post procedure

Patient

- Offer the patient hand-washing facilities.

Equipment/Environment

- Measure urine if appropriate and then discard safely.
- Discard the urinal or clean it as per local policy and return it to the patient for future use.

Nurse

- Remove gloves and apron and wash hands.
- Record amount on fluid balance chart (where applicable) (see page 159).

Points for practice

1. If the patient is sitting on or standing beside the bed, make sure the bed is at a suitable height and the brakes are on.

Preparation

Patient

• Explain any activities that may be required of the patient.

Equipment/Environment

• Fluid balance chart.
• Measuring jug.

Nurse

• Gloves should be worn when handling body fluids.

Procedure

1. All oral, intravenous and nasogastric intake should be recorded on the fluid intake side of the fluid balance chart (Figure 8.4). If continuous bladder irrigation is in progress, this should also be recorded (see page 195).
2. Record on the output section all urine output, diarrhoea or stoma output, nasogastric aspiration and vomit. Any other output that can be measured or weighed (e.g. wound drainage) should also be recorded.
3. The sections labelled 'Other' should be annotated according to individual patient requirements.
4. Patients who are independent in meeting their oral needs should be asked to note the nature and quantity of their oral fluid intake **PFP1,2**. If the patient is not independent, the nurse must do this.
5. Patients who are independent in meeting elimination needs will often be able to measure and chart their own urine output. If they are unable to do this themselves, provide them with a clearly labelled jug to leave in the sluice/toilet area.
6. Assess individual needs and monitor and record input and output at regular intervals.
7. A new chart will be needed for each 24-hour period. The fluid intake and output for the previous day is then totalled and the balance is calculated **PFP3,4**.

Fluid balance chart

Hospital/Ward: ST. SWITHINS   Date: 01.01.04

Hospital number: 1234567

Surname: SMITH   Forenames: FRANK

Date of birth: 01.01.1949   Sex: MALE

	Fluid intake			Fluid output			
Time (hrs)	Oral	IV	Other (specify route)	Urine	Vomit	Other (specify)	
01.00	NBM	B/F 500				WOUND DRAIN	
02.00		N/SALINE 0.9%					
03.00							
04.00							
05.00		↓					
06.00		5% Dex		400	90		
07.00		1000					
08.00							
09.00	↓						
10.00	30 H$_2$O						
11.00	30 H$_2$O						
12.00	30 H$_2$O			500			
13.00	30 H$_2$O						
14.00	30 H$_2$O						
15.00	30 H$_2$O						
16.00	30 H$_2$O						
17.00	30 H$_2$O	↓					
18.00	60 H$_2$O	5% Dex		450			
19.00	60 H$_2$O	1000					
20.00	60 H$_2$O						
21.00	60 H$_2$O						
22.00	100 TEA						
23.00							
24.00		↓		350	50		
TOTAL	580mls	2000		1800	140		

KEY:
NBM = NIL BY MOUTH
B/F = BROUGHT FORWARD

ALL MEASURMENTS IN MILLILITRES (MLS.)
TOTAL INPUT   =   580 + 2000 = 2580 MLS.
TOTAL OUTPUT = 1800 + 140 = 1940 MLS.
                 BALANCE = +640 MLS.

Figure 8.4 Example of a fluid balance chart

Points for practice

1. If the patient is on a fluid restriction (e.g. in renal failure), all oral fluid – including, for example, any milk with cereal – has to be recorded.

2. Accurate recording of intake and output is vital to be able to calculate the fluid balance. Gaps in recording (e.g. if the patient has been to theatre or for a test) make the balance inaccurate. In acute situations it may be necessary to measure the urine output every hour.

3. If there is more intake than output, the patient is in a positive fluid balance. If there is more output than intake, the patient is in a negative fluid balance.

4. In some patients, especially renal patients who do not pass urine, fluid balance is monitored by weighing the patient. Changes in weight will reflect fluid loss or gain.

Preparation

Patient

- Explain the procedure to gain consent and co-operation.
- Ensure privacy and dignity.

Equipment/Environment

- Penile sheath with adhesive.
- Catheter drainage bag (may be a leg bag if appropriate).
- Warm water, soap, disposable washcloth and towel.

Nurse

- Hands must be clean and an apron and gloves should be worn.

Procedure

1. Assist the patient into a supine position.
2. Prepare the catheter drainage bag.
3. Expose the patient's genitalia and place the penis gently on a towel.
4. Gently grasp the shaft of the penis. If the patient has not been circumcised, retract the foreskin.
5. Wash the tip of the penis at the urethral meatus and work outwards.
6. Wash the shaft of the penis in a downward stroke.
7. Repeat until the penis is clean, then rinse and dry gently.
8. Ensure the foreskin is returned to its normal position.
9. Clip hair at the base of the penis if this is likely to prevent the adhesive sticking.
10. Grasp the penis along the shaft. With your other hand, hold the rolled penile sheath at the tip of the penis and roll it halfway up the penis.
11. Attach the adhesive strip according to manufacturer's instructions and then roll the sheath over it to secure it into position (Figure 8.5). Make sure that the adhesive is not encircling the penis too tightly.
12. Attach the drainage tubing making sure the tip of the sheath is not twisted.

Post procedure

Patient

- Ensure patient is comfortable.
- Readjust clothing/bedclothes as necessary.

Equipment/Environment

- Dispose of clinical waste appropriately.
- Observe for leakage from the bag/tubing.

Nurse

- Remove gloves and apron and wash hands.
- Document application sheath, noting the condition of the penile skin.
- Check skin integrity at least once daily when attending to patient hygiene.

171

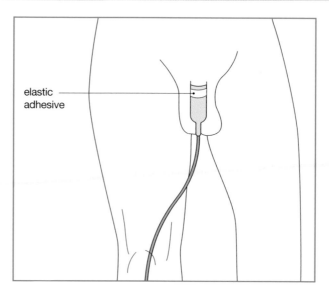

Figure 8.5 Penile sheath in position

Preparation

Patient

• Explain the procedure.

Equipment/Environment

• Clean container/jug for the urine **PFP1** .

Nurse

• Hands must be clean and gloves worn.
• An apron should be worn if there is a risk of splashing.

Procedure

1. Ask the patient to provide a urine sample.
2. If necessary, transfer the specimen to a clear container or jug.
3. Observe the urine for colour, concentration, odour and the presence of particles **PFP2** .

Post procedure

Patient

• Answer any questions.

Equipment/Environment

• Dispose of urine safely.
• Clean or dispose of the container/jug according to local policy.

Nurse

• Document urine observation and report any abnormalities.

Points for practice

1. A clear container or jug should be used if possible to enable the colour and clarity of the urine (i.e. presence of particles) to be assessed.

2. Normal urine is light yellow (straw coloured). A dark-yellow colour indicates that it is more concentrated than normal. The urine should be clear with no particles present. A malodorous or 'fishy' smell may indicate a urine infection. Any blood in the urine should always be reported, although if the patient is a woman, menstruation may be the cause.

Preparation

Patient

- Ask the patient to provide a urine specimen, or obtain a specimen, e.g. catheter specimen.

Equipment/Environment

- Fresh urine specimen in clean container/jug.
- Urine reagent sticks.
- Watch with a second-hand.

Nurse

- The hands should be clean and gloves should be worn.
- An apron should be worn if there is a risk of splashing.

Procedure

1. Check the expiry date of the reagent sticks and make sure that you are familiar with the manufacturer's instructions for use.
2. Remove a stick, making sure that you do not touch the coloured reagent pads with your hands. Replace the lid **PFP1**.
3. Dip the stick into the urine so that the reagent pads are completely immersed. Tap the stick against the side of the container/jug to remove excess urine.
4. Note the time on your watch. Accurate timing is crucial.
5. When the correct period of time has elapsed, read off the results by holding the stick alongside (but not touching) the pot and comparing the colour of each reagent pad with those displayed on the side (Figure 8.6). Make a mental note of the results **PFP2**.

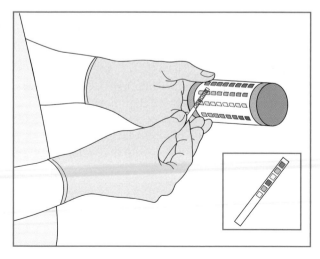

Figure 8.6 Urine testing

Urine reagent sticks commonly test for the following:

1. Specific gravity (normal range 1005–1030).
2. pH (normal range 4.5–8.0).
3. Protein, glucose, ketones, blood and bilirubin. All of these are negative in normal urine. The presence of these abnormalities might indicate the following (Baillie 2001):
   - Protein (proteinuria) – urinary tract infection.
   - Glucose (glycosuria) – diabetes mellitus or sometimes in pregnancy.
   - Ketones (ketonuria) – excessive fat metabolism due to diabetic ketoacidosis, vomiting or severe dieting.
   - Blood (haematuria) – kidney disorders (e.g. glomerulonephritis) or disorders of the urinary tract (e.g. kidney stones, tumours, infection).
   - Bilirubin – liver disease (e.g. hepatitis) or biliary tract obstruction (e.g. gall stones, carcinoma of the head of pancreas).

Post procedure

Patient

- Discuss the result with the patient as appropriate.

Equipment/Environment

- Discard the used stick in the clinical waste and dispose of the urine safely.
- Clean or dispose of the container/jug according to local policy.

Nurse

- Remove gloves and wash hands.
- Document urinalysis and report any abnormalities.

Points for practice

1. The lid of the reagent-sticks pot must always be replaced immediately after use to prevent moisture getting in.

2. Make a mental note of the results or if necessary jot them down on a piece of paper. Do not take the patient's charts into the sluice to prevent contamination or splashing with water.

Preparation

Patient

- Explain the procedure, to gain consent and co-operation.
- Ensure the patient's privacy and dignity are maintained.
- Urine specimens should be collected as soon as possible after waking.

Equipment/Environment

- Toilet, urinal or bedpan.
- Universal specimen pot.
- Gauze swabs, soap and water.
- Paper towels.

Nurse

- Gloves should be worn if assisting with the procedure.

Procedure

Male patient

1. Instruct/assist the patient to retract the foreskin and clean the skin surrounding the urethral meatus with soap and water, using each gauze swab only once. Dry with paper towels.
2. Ask the patient to start urinating into the urinal/toilet then stop, pass the middle part of the stream into the specimen pot (10ml is sufficient) and then finish urinating into the urinal/toilet **PFP1**.

Female patient

1. Instruct/assist the patient to clean the urethral meatus with soap and water, using each gauze swab only once. Swab from front to back. Dry with paper towels.
2. Ask the patient to start urinating into the urinal/toilet then stop, pass the middle part of the stream into the specimen pot (10ml is sufficient) and then finish urinating into the urinal/toilet **PFP1**.

Post procedure

Patient

- Offer the patient hand-washing facilities.
- Ensure the patient is comfortable.

Equipment/Environment

- Discard all waste appropriately.

Nurse

- Ensure the specimen pot is securely closed
- Remove gloves and wash hands.
- Complete patient details on the label **PFP2**. Place in a plastic specimen bag with the pathology request form (Figure 8.7).

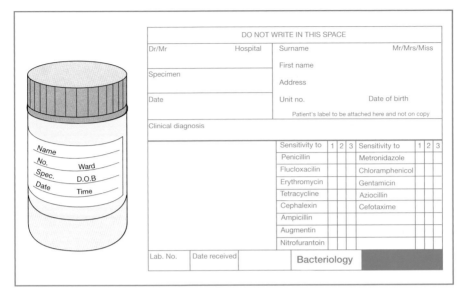

Figure 8.7 Urine specimen and request form

- Place the specimen in the refrigerator for dispatch to the laboratory as soon as possible.
- Document the date and time of specimen collection in the nursing records.

Points for practice

1. Some specimen pots for midstream urine sample have a special funnel attached to facilitate collection. This is removed and discarded before the specimen is sent to the laboratory.

2. The patient's details should include: surname; first name; date of birth; hospital number; ward; and type of specimen (i.e. MSU).

Preparation

Patient

- Explain the procedure, to gain consent and co-operation.
- Maintain dignity and privacy throughout the procedure.

Equipment/Environment

- Disposable gloves.
- Alcohol-impregnated swab.
- Non-toothed 'gate' clamp **PFP1**.
- A 20ml syringe **PFP2**.
- Universal specimen container.

Nurse

- Hands must be washed and dried thoroughly.
- An apron and gloves should be worn.

Procedure

1. If there is no urine present in the catheter tubing, clamp it below the sampling port 15–20 minutes before collecting the sample, to allow urine to collect.
2. Clean the sampling port on the tubing with the alcohol-impregnated swab and allow to dry.
3. Insert the syringe into the sampling port and aspirate the required amount of urine **PFP3**. If a needle is required, take care not to go right through the tubing and out the other side.
4. Transfer the urine to the specimen pot and replace the lid securely **PFP4**.

Post procedure

Patient

- Ensure the patient is comfortable.

Equipment/Environment

- Discard clinical waste and sharps appropriately.
- If used, remove the clamp from the tubing to allow free drainage.

Nurse

- Remove gloves and apron and wash hands.
- Label the specimen **PFP5** and place it in a plastic specimen bag with the laboratory request form.
- Place the specimen in the refrigerator for dispatch to the laboratory as soon as possible.
- Document the date and time of specimen collection in the nursing records.

Points for practice

1. It is important that a non-toothed clamp is used to prevent damage to the tubing.

2. Most catheter bags have a 'needle-free' sampling port, which allows the syringe to be connected without the need for a needle. If a needle is required, an orange needle (25G) should be used.

3. A 10ml sample of urine is usually sufficient.

4. If a needle has been used, remove it from the syringe before transferring the specimen, in case it falls into the pot and contaminates the specimen.

5. The patient's details should include: surname; first name; date of birth; hospital number; ward; and date, time and type of specimen (i.e. CSU).

Preparation

Patient

- Explain the procedure, and assess the patient's ability to participate in obtaining the collection.

Equipment/Environment

- Toilet/urinal/bedpan as required and jug.
- A 24-hour urine collection container (more than one may be required).
- Bed/door sign indicating 24-hour urine collection is in progress, time started and when due to be completed.

Nurse

- Gloves should be worn when handling urine.

Procedure

1. Label the container clearly with the patient's name, hospital number and ward.
2. When urine is next passed, discard it. The 24-hour period begins at this point.
3. Every time the patient passes urine, it is collected and placed in the container, which is stored in the sluice **PFP1** .
4. If the patient is undertaking collection independently, check compliance and continued understanding.
5. Ask/assist the patient to empty their bladder just before the end of the 24-hour collection period.

Post procedure

Patient

- Advise the patient when the 24-hour period is completed.

Equipment/Environment

- Remove sign from the bed/door.
- Clean or discard the jug according to local policy.

Nurse

- Record completion time of test.
- Ensure that the urine collection and laboratory request form are sent to the laboratory as soon as possible.

Points for practice

1. Should a sample of urine become contaminated or accidentally be discarded, the test must be terminated and restarted.

Preparation

Patient

- Provide a clear explanation of the collection procedure and the need for three consecutive early morning specimens **PFP1**.

Equipment/Environment

- Universal specimen pot.
- Gauze swabs, soap and water.
- Paper towels.

Nurse

- Gloves should be worn if the patient requires assistance.

Procedure

1. Ask/assist female patients to clean and dry the vulval area around the urinary meatus, using wet gauze swabs and paper towels. Ask male patients to retract the foreskin and clean and dry the end of the penis.
2. Ask/assist the patient to hold the specimen pot in a gloved hand and pass **the beginning and the end** of the stream of urine into the pot **PFP2**. The middle of the stream should be passed into the lavatory, bedpan or urinal.
3. If the patient is unable to stop and start the stream of urine, the bladder should be emptied completely into a sterile container and a small portion (10–20ml) of that amount put into the specimen pot.
4. Repeat the procedure on the next two consecutive days.

Post procedure

Patient

- The patient may be unaware of the possible diagnosis.
- Deal with the patient's questions with sensitivity.

Equipment/Environment

- Ensure the specimen pot is securely closed. Label the pot **PFP3** and place in a plastic specimen bag with the laboratory request form. Refrigerate until dispatch to the laboratory.

Nurse

- Document the date and time of specimen collection in the nursing records.

Points for practice

1. A urine specimen for cytology is requested when a malignancy is suspected. The patient may not be aware of this at this point and care must be taken to avoid unnecessary alarm.

2. The first part and end of the stream of urine are collected as these are most likely to contain malignant cells if present in the bladder.

3. The patient's details should include: surname; first name; date of birth; hospital number and ward. Each specimen must also be clearly labelled with the date and time, and numbered 1, 2 or 3 to ensure the correct order is known in the laboratory.

Procedure

This specimen is collected in the same way as a specimen for cytology (see page 181) except that only the first part of the stream of urine is required.

Preparation

Patient

- Explain the procedure, to gain consent and co-operation.
- Ensure the patient's privacy and dignity are maintained throughout.
- Ask/assist the patient to wash the perineal area and dry thoroughly.

Equipment/Environment

- Clean trolley or other appropriate surface.
- Sterile catheterisation pack `PFP1`.
- Two urinary catheters of appropriate size `PFP2`.
- Sachet of sterile 0.9% sodium chloride.
- Catheter bag with stand/holder.
- Lubricant/anaesthetic gel.
- Universal specimen container.
- A 10ml syringe and 10ml ampoule of sterile water.
- Disposable waterproof absorbent pad.
- Alcohol hand-rub or hand-washing facilities.
- Good light source.

Nurse

- Wash and dry hands thoroughly.
- An apron should be worn.
- Two nurses may be necessary if the patient requires assistance to adopt the required position.

Procedure

1. Take the prepared trolley to the patient's bedside and position it on the right or left depending on the nurse's dominant hand.
2. Raise the bed to an appropriate height and ensure a good light source.
3. Ask/assist the patient to adopt a supine position with knees flexed and thighs relaxed to externally rotate the hip joints. If the patient is unable to adopt this position, she can be assisted onto her side with her upper leg flexed at the hip and knee.
4. Arrange the bedclothes to expose the genital area, and place the disposable pad beneath the buttocks.
5. Wash your hands or clean them with alcohol hand-rub.
6. Ensuring principles of asepsis are maintained, open the catheterisation pack and any additional packs and equipment.
7. Open the catheter but do not remove it from its internal wrapping, and place it in the sterile receiver on the trolley. Expose the tip of the catheter by pulling off the top of the wrapper at the serrated edge.
8. Pour the sachet of 0.9% sodium chloride into the gallipot.
9. Open the catheter bag and arrange it at the side of the bed, ensuring that the catheter connection is easily accessible and remains sterile.
10. Squeeze a small amount of lubricant or anaesthetic gel onto a gauze swab `PFP3`

11. Draw up the amount of sterile water required to inflate the balloon (PFP4)
12. Wash your hands or clean them with alcohol-based rub, and put on the sterile gloves (PFP5).
13. Place sterile dressing towels onto the bed area between the patient's legs and over the patient's thighs.
14. Using a gauze swab and your non-dominant hand, retract the labia minora to expose the urethral meatus (Figure 8.8). This hand should be used to maintain labial separation until catheterisation has been completed.
15. Clean the perineal area with 0.9% sodium chloride, using a new gauze swab for each stroke and cleaning from the front towards the anus.
16. Place the receiver holding the catheter, on the sterile towel between the patient's legs.
17. Lubricate the catheter tip with lubricating gel.
18. Holding the catheter so that the distal end remains in the receiver and gradually advancing it out of its wrapper, introduce the catheter into the urethra in an upward and backward direction for approximately 5–7cm or until urine flows out of the catheter end. Advance the catheter a further 5cm. Do not force the catheter (PFP6).
19. Inflate the balloon with the correct amount of water (see Figure 8.11).
20. Place a small amount of urine (10–20ml) into the specimen pot (PFP7).
21. Attach the catheter drainage bag and position it so that there is no pulling on the catheter.

Post procedure

Patient

- Make sure the patient is dry and comfortable.
- If the patient's condition allows, encourage oral fluids.

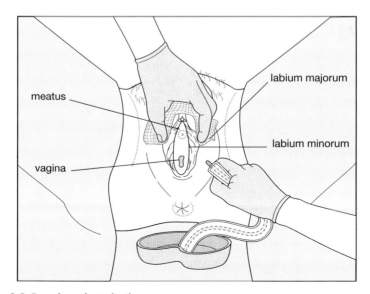

Figure 8.8 Female catheterisation

Equipment/Environment

- Dispose of equipment and clinical waste appropriately.

Nurse

- Measure and record the amount of urine contained in the receiver.
- Remove gloves and apron and wash hands.
- Document catheterisation in the nursing records.
- Monitor urine output as appropriate.
- Send the specimen, with the request form, to the laboratory as soon as possible, for culture and sensitivity testing.

Points for practice

1. A catheterisation pack contains the following sterile items: kidney dish/receiver, dressing towels, gloves, gallipot and gauze swabs. If a catheterisation pack is not available, a sterile dressing pack containing gloves should be used and the other items added as required.

2. When choosing the size of catheter to be inserted, choose the smallest size possible. For most women a 12FG or 14FG will be adequate, although a larger size may be necessary if there is blood or sediment in the urine. A second catheter is useful in case catheterisation is unsuccessful with the first. There are catheters available with a shorter shaft length (23cm). These reduce the risk of kinking and looping and so allow more efficient drainage, and can also be more easily concealed if being used with a leg bag. However, they are not suitable for all women.

3. If anaesthetic gel is used, this should be inserted into the urethra 5 minutes prior to catheter insertion.

4. A balloon size of 10ml is common, as this is usually sufficient to retain the catheter. Larger balloon sizes may irritate the bladder and cause bladder spasm. It is important to use the exact amount of water indicated on the catheter.

5. Concerns about contamination of the hands during urethral cleansing and instillation of gel can be overcome by using two pairs of sterile gloves (one on top of the other) at the start of the procedure. The outer pair can then be removed after cleansing, prior to catheter insertion.

6. If the catheter is accidentally inserted into the vagina, leave it in place to prevent it happening again, and use a new catheter. Once this is successfully in place, remove the first catheter from the vagina.

7. Urine from the sterile receiver or contained within the plastic wrapper can be tipped into the specimen pot.

Preparation

Patient

- Explain the procedure, to gain consent and co-operation.
- Ensure the patient's privacy and dignity are maintained throughout.
- Ask/assist the patient to wash the penis and perineal area and dry thoroughly.

Equipment/Environment

- Clean trolley or other appropriate surface.
- Sterile catheterisation pack **PFP1** .
- Two urinary catheters of an appropriate size **PFP2** .
- Sterile anaesthetic lubricating gel in syringe/tube applicator.
- Sachet of sterile 0.9% sodium chloride.
- A 10ml syringe and 10ml ampoule of sterile water.
- Catheter drainage bag and stand/holder.
- Universal specimen container.
- Alcohol hand-rub or hand-washing facilities.
- Waterproof absorbent pad.
- Good light source.

Nurse

- Wash and dry hands thoroughly.
- An apron should be worn.
- Two nurses may be necessary if the patient needs assistance to adopt the required position **PFP3** .

Procedure

1. Take the prepared trolley to the patient's bedside and position it on the right or left depending on the nurse's dominant hand.
2. Raise the bed to an appropriate height and ensure a good light source.
3. Ask/assist the patient to adopt a supine position with the legs extended.
4. Arrange the bedclothes to expose the genital area, and place the absorbent pad underneath the buttocks.
5. Wash your hands or clean them with alcohol hand-rub.
6. Ensuring the principles of asepsis are maintained, open the catheterisation pack and any additional packs and equipment.
7. Open the catheter but do not remove it from its inner wrapper, and place it in the sterile receiver on the trolley. Expose the tip of the catheter by pulling off the top of the wrapper at the serrated edge.
8. Pour the sachet of 0.9% sodium chloride into the gallipot.
9. Draw up the amount of sterile water required to inflate the balloon **PFP4** .
10. Open the catheter drainage bag and arrange it at the side of the bed, ensuring the attachment tip is easily accessible and remains sterile.
11. Wash your hands or clean them with alcohol hand-rub. Put on the sterile gloves **PFP5** .
12. Tear a hole in the centre of the sterile towel. Cover the patient's abdomen and thighs with the towel, with the penis protruding through the hole.

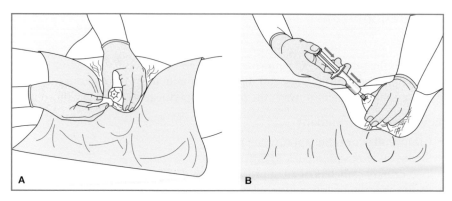

Figure 8.9 A = Cleaning the glans penis.
B = Instilling the anaesthetic gel

13. Attach the nozzle to the anaesthetic lubricating gel.
14. With your non-dominant hand and using a piece of sterile gauze, grasp the shaft of the penis and retract the foreskin.
15. Clean the glans penis with the sterile 0.9% sodium chloride, ensuring the tips of the fingers remain sterile (Figure 8.9A).
16. Still holding the penis, insert the nozzle of the anaesthetic lubricating gel into the urethra and instill the gel into the urethra (Figure 8.9B).
17. Massage the gel along the urethra and wait 5 minutes for it to act.
18. Grasp the shaft of the penis with your non-dominant hand and hold the penis upwards, to extend the peno-scrotal flexure.
19. Expose the tip of the catheter by pulling off the top of the wrapper at the serrated edge. Replace it in the sterile receiver.
20. Place the receiver containing the catheter, between the patient's thighs.
21. With your dominant hand holding and gradually withdrawing the wrapper, insert the catheter 15–25cm into the urethra until urine flows (Figure 8.10). If resistance is met at the external sphincter, extend the penis further towards the abdomen. Ask the patient to cough or strain gently as if passing urine. If resistance continues, do not force the catheter: stop the procedure and seek medical advice.
22. When urine is flowing, advance the catheter further, to ensure the catheter is in the bladder.
23. Inflate the balloon with the correct amount of sterile water (Figure 8.11).
24. Place a small amount of urine (10–20ml) into the specimen pot.
25. Attach the catheter drainage bag and position it so that it is well supported to prevent traction on the catheter.
26. Replace the foreskin.

Post procedure

Patient

• Ensure the patient is dry and comfortable.
• If the patient's condition allows, encourage oral fluids.

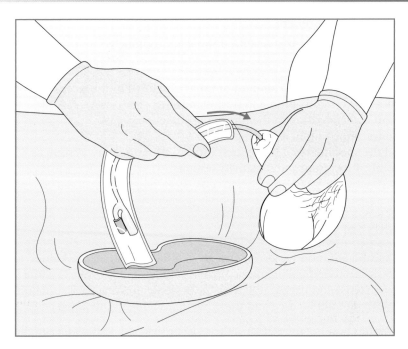

Figure 8.10 Inserting the catheter

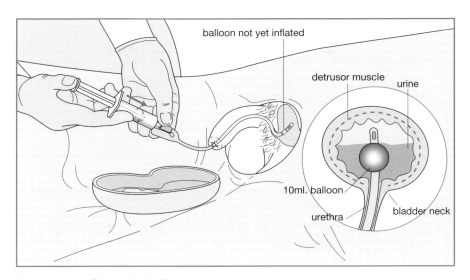

balloon not yet inflated

detrusor muscle

urine

10ml. balloon

urethra

bladder neck

Figure 8.11 Inflating the balloon

Equipment/Environment

- Dispose of equipment and clinical waste appropriately.

Nurse

- Measure and record the amount of urine contained in the receiver.
- Remove gloves and apron and wash hands.
- Record catheterisation in the nursing documentation.
- Monitor urine output as appropriate.
- Send the specimen and the request form to the laboratory as soon as possible, for culture and sensitivity testing.

Points for practice

1. A catheterisation pack contains the following sterile items: kidney dish/receiver, dressing towels, gloves, gallipot and gauze swabs. If a catheterisation pack is not available, a sterile dressing pack containing gloves should be used and the other items added as required.

2. When choosing the size of catheter to be inserted, choose the smallest size possible. For most men a 12FG or 14FG will be adequate, although a larger size may be necessary if there is blood or sediment in the urine. Trauma from catheter insertion is commonly associated with urethral stricture formation. Trauma arises when too large a catheter is used, when the catheter is forced on insertion or when the balloon is inflated in the urethra. Necrosis in the bladder neck may also result from an overly large catheter or balloon. A second catheter is useful in case catheterisation is unsuccessful with the first.

3. In most hospitals, only registered nurses who have received additional training may perform male catheterisation.

4. A balloon size of 10ml is recommended, as this is usually sufficient to retain the catheter. Larger balloon sizes may irritate the bladder and cause bladder spasm and bypassing of urine (a 30ml balloon is used as a haemostat following urological procedures and should not be used for routine catheterisation). It is important to use the exact amount of water indicated on the catheter.

5. Concerns about contamination of the hands during urethral cleansing and instillation of gel can be overcome by using two pairs of sterile gloves (one on top of the other) at the start of the procedure. The outer pair can then be removed after cleansing, prior to catheter insertion.

Preparation

Patient

- Explain the procedure, to gain consent and co-operation PFP1 .
- Ensure the patient's privacy and dignity are maintained.
- Place the patient in a supine position with knees and hips flexed and slightly apart.

Equipment/Environment

- Soap, water, disposable washcloth, clean towel.

Nurse

- Wash and dry hands thoroughly.
- Put on apron and gloves.

Procedure

Female patients

1. Clean the vulval area from above downward using warm soapy water PFP2,3 .
2. Clean the catheter by gently wiping in one direction away from the catheter–meatal junction. Rinse well PFP4 .
3. Dry the area by patting with a towel.

Male patients

1. Retract the foreskin before cleaning PFP2,3 .
2. Clean the shaft of the catheter away from the catheter–meatal junction and rinse well PFP4 .
3. Dry the area by patting with a towel.
4. Replace the foreskin on completion of cleaning.

Post procedure

Patient

- Ensure the patient is dry and comfortable.

Equipment/Environment

- Dispose of all waste appropriately.

Nurse

- Remove gloves and apron and wash hands.
- Record catheter care and report any abnormalities.

Points for practice

1. Where possible, patients should be taught to attend to their own meatal and perineal hygiene, thus reducing the risk of cross-infection. Powders or lotions should not be used after cleansing as these trap organisms in the area.

2. The main aim of cleansing is to remove secretions and encrustation and prevent infection. Cleansing with soap and water has been shown to be as effective as any other method; however, in some hospitals clean swabs and 0.9% sodium chloride solution are used.

3. Perineal and meatal hygiene should be performed once daily unless there is excessive exudate or encrustation.

4. Supra-pubic catheters are inserted through the abdominal wall, directly into the bladder. The insertion site should be treated as a surgical wound (see page 222).

Preparation

Patient

- Explain the procedure to the patient although it should not cause any discomfort.
- The patient may prefer the bed to be screened.

Equipment/Environment

- Measuring jug **PFP1** and paper towel to cover.
- Tissue or alcohol-impregnated swab.

Nurse

- Wash and dry hands thoroughly.
- Gloves and an apron should be worn.

Procedure

1. Take the covered jug and other equipment to the bedside.
2. If the drainage bag is on a floor stand, it does not need to be removed from the stand for emptying. If the bag is hanging on the side of the bed, it may need to be removed from its holder. Hold the bag over or balance it on the top of the jug, making sure that the drainage port does not touch the jug (Figure 8.12).
3. Open the drainage port and allow the urine to flow into the jug. Close the drainage port.
4. Wipe the aperture with the alcohol-impregnated swab or tissue to prevent dripping.
5. Reposition the catheter bag as necessary to ensure that the drainage port is not touching the floor and the tubing is not kinked, to allow free drainage into the bag.
6. Cover the jug and take it to the sluice. Measure the amount of urine and discard **PFP2** .

Post procedure

Patient

- If the patient's condition allows, encourage oral fluids.

Equipment/Environment

- Clean or discard the urine jug according to local policy **PFP3** .

Nurse

- Remove gloves and apron and wash hands.
- Record amount on fluid balance chart if appropriate.

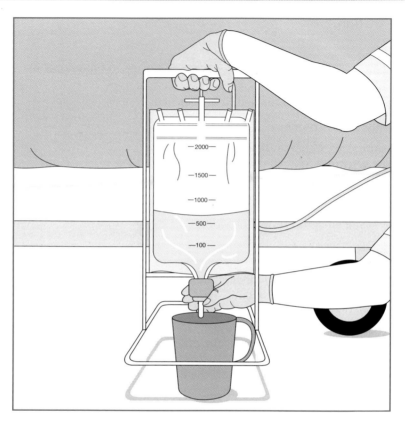

Figure 8.12 Emptying the catheter bag

Points for practice

1. The jug used will be one that is only used for urine. This will usually be a different colour or design from those used for drinking water.

2. If hourly urine measurement is required, a special drainage bag is used which incorporates a small reservoir that can be emptied into the drainage bag without opening the 'closed' system.

3. The cleaning of the jug will vary according to local policy. If disposable, it will be discarded. If not disposable, it may be placed in the bedpan washer or returned to the sterile supplies department for decontamination.

Preparation

Patient

- Explain the procedure, to gain consent and co-operation.
- Ensure the patient's privacy and dignity are maintained.
- The patient will be catheterised with a three-way urethral catheter.

Equipment/Environment

- Clean trolley or other appropriate surface.
- Sterile dressing pack containing gloves.
- Sterile dressing towel.
- Antiseptic skin-cleansing solution according to local policy.
- Non-toothed clamp.
- Sterile jug.
- Sterile 'Y' shaped irrigation set and fluid as prescribed (usually 0.9% sodium chloride) at room temperature **PFP1** .
- Infusion stand **PFP2** .
- Large catheter drainage bag
- Alcohol hand rub.

Nurse

- Wash and dry hands thoroughly.
- An apron should be worn.

Procedure

1. Take the trolley and equipment to the bedside.
2. Open the irrigation fluid bags and hang on the infusion stand.
3. Maintaining asepsis, attach and prime the irrigation set to expel all air. Close the flow control clamp of the irrigation set **PFP3** .
4. Ask/assist the patient to adopt a supine position, and expose the catheter and catheter drainage tube.
5. Clamp the catheter using a non-toothed clamp or the clamp on the catheter-bag tubing (Figure 8.13) **PFP4** .
6. Wash and dry your hands.
7. Maintaining asepsis, open the dressing pack and other equipment, attach the disposal bag to the side of the trolley and pour antiseptic solution into the gallipot.
8. Cleanse your hands with alcohol hand rub, allow to dry and then put on the sterile gloves.
9. Place the sterile towel underneath the irrigation inlet of the catheter.
10. Remove and discard the spigot from the irrigation port of the catheter.
11. Thoroughly clean around the irrigation port with antiseptic solution, using each swab only once and wiping in the same direction.
12. Maintaining asepsis, attach the irrigation set to the irrigation port but do not open the flow control clamp.

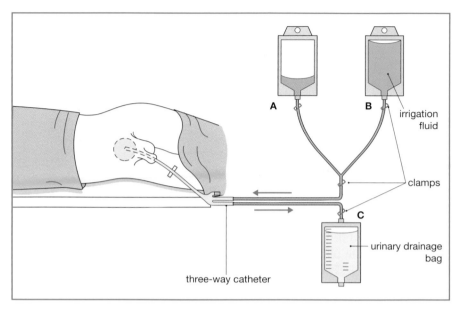

Figure 8.13 Continuous bladder irrigation

13. Release the clamp on the catheter and allow accumulated urine to drain. Empty the contents of the catheter bag into the sterile jug (see page 193).
14. Discard gloves.
15. Open the flow control clamp and set irrigation at the prescribed rate, ensuring that fluid/urine is draining freely into the catheter bag **PFP5** (Figure 8.13).

Post procedure

Patient

- Assist the patient into a comfortable position.
- Advise the patient to report any bladder distension, pain or discomfort **PFP6**.

Equipment/Environment

- Dispose of equipment and waste appropriately.
- Measure urine and discard **PFP7**.

Nurse

- Remove apron and wash hands.
- Record the time of commencement and the volume of irrigation fluid being infused on the fluid balance chart.
- Check the volume in the catheter drainage bag at least every hour for the first 24 hours, empty as necessary and record on fluid balance chart.

Points for practice

1. Three-litre bags of irrigation solution are preferable, as they require less frequent changing and interruption of the closed system.

2. Irrigation fluid should be suspended from a separate infusion stand from that used for intravenous infusions.

3. When priming the irrigation set, make sure that only one clamp (e.g. A or B Figure 8.13) is open. This will prevent irrigation fluid running from one bottle to the other.

4. It is important to use a non-toothed clamp to prevent damage to the tubing.

5. The rate of infusion will vary according to the degree of haematuria. The aim is to obtain drainage fluid that is rosé in colour. Haematuria will be greatest in the first 12 hours following surgery and 6–9L of irrigation fluid is likely to be required. This should fall to 3–6L in the second 12 hours. Only one bag of irrigation fluid is used at a time. When the first bag is empty the second bag can be commenced immediately ensuring continuous flow. In the meantime, the empty bag can be replaced.

6. If clot retention is suspected (the output stops and the patient complains of pain and discomfort) irrigation should be stopped immediately and the problem reported. A bladder washout may be required (see page 198).

7. The volume of irrigation fluid being infused and the amount of drainage in the catheter bag should be recorded on the fluid balance chart. The difference between the two figures is the urine output (Table 8.1).

Table 8.1 Example of irrigation-fluid and urine-output charting.

Irrigation-Fluid and Urine Output Charting		
Irrigation	**Irrigation Output**	**Difference = Urine**
3000	1050	
	950	
	1250	
	Total = 3250ml	= 3250ml (Output)
		−3000ml (Input)
		= 250ml URINE

Preparation

Patient

- Explain the procedure, to gain consent and co-operation.
- Ensuring dignity and privacy are maintained, position the patient to allow access to the catheter.
- An absorbent, waterproof pad should be placed under the patient's buttocks.

Equipment/Environment

- Clean trolley or other appropriate surface.
- Sterile dressing pack containing gloves.
- Sterile dressing towel.
- A 50ml or 60ml bladder tip syringe **PFP1**.
- Sterile jug.
- Sterile washout solution as prescribed (most commonly 0.9% sodium chloride) at room temperature.
- Two sterile bowls or receivers.
- Antiseptic cleansing solution according to local policy.
- Alcohol hand-rub or hand-washing facilities.
- Non-toothed clamp.
- Sterile spigot if washout solution is to be retained.
- New catheter drainage bag.

Nurse

- Wash and dry hands thoroughly.
- An apron should be worn.

Procedure

1. Take the prepared trolley to the patient's bedside and position it on the right or left depending on the nurse's dominant hand.
2. Maintaining asepsis, open the sterile dressing pack and additional equipment including the sterile jug, bladder syringe and sterile bowls/receivers. Pour antiseptic solution into the gallipot. Pour washout solution into the jug.
3. Open the catheter drainage bag and place it in an accessible position, leaving the cover on the catheter connector to maintain sterility.
4. Arrange the bed clothes to expose the genital area and check the absorbent pad is under the buttocks.
5. Wash and dry your hands or clean them using alcohol hand-rub, and put on the sterile gloves.
6. Draw up 30–40ml of washout fluid into the syringe (note the amount) and expel the air **PFP2**.
7. Place the sterile towel between the patient's legs, creating a sterile field.
8. Place one receiver on the sterile towel.
9. Clamp the catheter.

10. Cover both the catheter and drainage tube with sterile gauze and touching only the gauze, disconnect the catheter from the tubing. Place the end of the catheter in the sterile receiver.
11. Clean the end of the catheter with antiseptic solution and attach the bladder syringe. Unclamp the catheter and gently instill the solution into the bladder (Figure 8.14).
12. Remove the syringe and allow the solution to drain out naturally into the second sterile receiver. If the solution does not drain, aspirate gently using the bladder syringe **PFP3**. Repeat the process, using 30–40ml of solution each time, until the urine is clear and flowing freely **PFP4**.
13. Connect the new drainage bag.

Post procedure

Patient

- Ensure the patient is comfortable and is not experiencing bladder discomfort.
- Encourage fluids and mobilisation.

Equipment/Environment

- Dispose of equipment and waste appropriately.

Nurse

- Remove gloves and apron and wash hands.
- Measure the input and output to calculate any urine output.
- Document bladder washout and report any abnormalities.

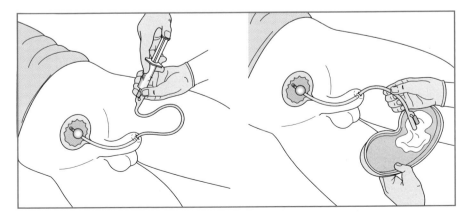

Figure 8.14 Instilling washout solution

Points for practice

1. A bladder-tip syringe differs from other syringes in that the tip is large and designed to fit the opening of a urinary catheter.

2. Some commercially prepared washout solutions may be attached directly onto the catheter and so do not require a syringe.

3. If no fluid is returned after instillation of the first 30ml, instill a further 30ml. If there is still no return, seek advice.

4. If the solution contains medication and is to be retained, the catheter should be spigoted for the prescribed length of time.

Preparation

Patient

- Explain the procedure, to gain consent and co-operation **PFP1**.
- Ensure the patient's privacy and dignity are maintained throughout.
- Position the patient in a supine position with knees and hips flexed and slightly apart.

Equipment/Environment

- Clean trolley or tray.
- A 20ml syringe **PFP2**.
- Large disposable absorbent pad.
- Receiver.
- Yellow waste bag for disposal of catheter and catheter bag.
- Specimen pot and 20ml syringe (for catheter specimen).

Nurse

- Choose appropriate time for catheter removal **PFP3**.
- Wash and dry hands thoroughly.
- An apron and gloves should be worn.

Procedure

1. Take the equipment to the bedside.
2. Take a catheter specimen of urine (see page 178).
3. Place the disposable pad under the buttocks and the receiver between the patient's thighs.
4. Check the volume of water in the balloon (usually written on the catheter), attach the syringe to the balloon port on the catheter and withdraw the water to deflate the balloon **PFP4**.
5. Ask the patient to breathe in and out. As the patient exhales, gently but firmly withdraw the catheter into the receiver.

Post procedure

Patient

- Assist the patient into a comfortable position and ensure a lavatory or urinal/commode is nearby.
- Advise the patient regarding the possibility of frequency, urgency, haematuria and dysuria **PFP5**.
- Advise the patient to increase oral fluid intake (2–2.5L in 24 hours).
- Ask the patient to inform the nurse when urine has been passed.

Equipment/Environment

- Dispose of equipment and waste appropriately.

Nurse

- Remove gloves and apron and wash hands.
- Record the amount of urine in the catheter drainage bag on the fluid balance chart.
- Document the time of catheter removal and when the patient subsequently passes urine.
- Label the catheter specimen and send it to the laboratory with the request form or refrigerate it as soon as possible.

Points for practice

1. The patient may be frightened of catheter removal and imagine it to be extremely painful.

2. The size of syringe required will depend on the amount of water in the catheter balloon. This is written on the catheter itself.

3. Traditionally, catheters have been removed first thing in the morning. However, research has shown that midnight removal increases the length of time before passing urine, leading to a greater initial volume. This is said to aid a faster return to normal voiding and a reduction in anxiety.

4. If problems are encountered when deflating the balloon or withdrawing the catheter, medical advice should be sought.

5. The patient may well experience feelings of wanting to pass urine following removal of the catheter. Male patients should be discouraged from placing a urinal in position 'just in case', as this may encourage frequent small volumes to be passed or 'dribbling'. A frequency chart may be requested for the first 24 hours. Haematuria (blood in the urine) may be the result of trauma following catheter removal and dysuria (pain when passing urine) may be due to inflammation of the urethra.

Principles

- Regular care and inspection of a stoma is vital so that any deterioration in the stoma, such as necrosis, retraction, or skin excoriation, is reported promptly. Delay exacerbates the problem and may cause pain and distress for the patient.
- Gloves and an apron should be worn when caring for a stoma.

Stoma bag

- Ensure that the flange of the bag is cut according to the template so that it fits snugly around the stoma (Figure 8.15). If the aperture is too small, the edge of the aperture will cause friction on the delicate blood vessels of the stoma, causing bruising or bleeding. If, on the other hand, the aperture is too big, the contents of the bowel will spill out of the stoma onto the surrounding skin, causing excoriation and soreness.
- When the bag is removed, it is important to do this gently so that the skin is not pulled. Use counter-pressure with your other hand.
- The skin and stoma should be cleaned whenever the bag is changed, to prevent skin soreness. A special stoma cream may be advocated if there are skin problems at the stoma site. Make sure the surrounding skin is dry before attaching a new bag.
- Ensure the bag is securely attached to the skin, thus preventing leakage and distress for the patient. Some stoma bags have a clip at the bottom to enable them to be emptied without removing the bag. Take care that the clip is securely fitted to prevent leakage.
- Many trusts have a stoma nurse specialist for advice regarding care of the stoma.

Preparation

Patient

- Assist the patient to sit or lie in a comfortable position **PFP1**.
- Ensure privacy and dignity are maintained throughout.
- Place a protective pad next to the stoma site to protect clothing.

Equipment/Environment

- Clean stoma bag and flange **PFP2**.
- Scissors to cut the flange or aperture of the bag to the correct size.
- Stoma template
- Tissues or gauze swabs.
- Jug to dispose of the contents of the used bag.
- Yellow clinical waste bag.
- Soap and water for cleansing the skin.
- Barrier cream if advised.

Nurse

- Wash and dry hands thoroughly.
- Put on apron and gloves.

Procedure

1. If the stoma bag is the type that can be emptied before removal, empty the contents of the stoma bag into the jug.
2. Gently peel the adhesive off the skin, using the other hand to apply counter-pressure.
3. Wipe the skin free of faeces and secretions using damp tissues or gauze.
4. Clean the skin and stoma using soap and water and dry well.
5. Check the condition of the stoma and the surrounding skin and apply barrier cream if appropriate.
6. Cut a hole to the correct size in the bag or flange using the stoma template as a guide.
7. Place the flange and/or the bag over the stoma so that the aperture fits snugly and is well attached (Figures 8.15 & 8.16).
8. If appropriate, attach the clip to the base of the bag **PFP3**.

Post procedure

Patient

- Offer the patient a hand wash if they have participated in the process.
- Ensure the patient is comfortable.

Equipment/Environment

- Dispose of excreta down the sluice.
- Discard the soiled bag and other clinical waste appropriately.
- Return unused equipment.

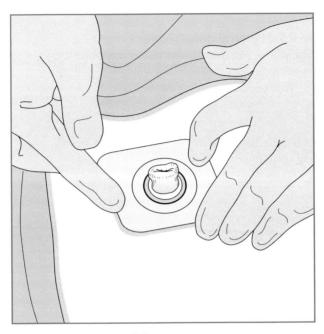

Figure 8.15 Fitting the flange around the stoma

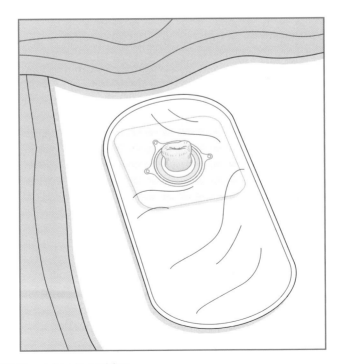

Figure 8.16 Stoma bag in position

Nurse

- Remove gloves and apron and wash hands.
- Document the stoma bag change and report any abnormalities.

Points for practice

1. Patients are usually taught to care for their own stomas. Many patients have a bag containing all the necessary equipment.

2. Some stoma bags have a separate flange and bag; others are one-piece appliances.

3. If the bag is the type that can be emptied without removing it, there will be a special 'roll-up' clip at the bottom. Take care not to discard this when emptying the bag.

Bibliography/Suggested reading

Allison M. Comparing methods of stoma function. *Nursing Standard* 1995, **9**(24):25–28.

Baillie L. *Developing practical nursing skills.* London: Arnold; 2001.

Black P. Choosing the correct stoma appliance. *British Journal of Nursing* 1994, **3**(11):545–550.

Black P. Practical stoma management. *Nursing Standard* 1997, **11**(47):49–55.

Brown J. Collecting midstream specimens of urine – the research base. *Nursing Times* 1991, **87**(13):49–52.

Cook R. Urinalysis: ensuring accurate urine testing. *Nursing Standard* 1996, **10**(46):49–52.

Daffurn K. Fluid balance charts: do they measure up? *British Journal of Nursing* 1994, **3**(16):816–820.

Department of Health. *The Essence of Care: continence and bladder and bowel care.* London: Department of Health, 2001.

Evans, A. Blocked urinary catheters: nurses' preventative role. *Nursing Times* 2001, **97**(1):37–38.

Evans, A, Godfrey, H. Bladder washouts in the management of long-term catheters. *British Journal of Nursing* 2000, **9**(14):900–906.

Getliffe, K. Review of catheter care guidelines. *Nursing Times* 2001, **97**(20):NT Plus, 70–71.

Godfrey H, Evans A. Catherization and urinary tract infections: microbiology. *British Journal of Nursing* 2000, **9**(11):682–690.

Gould D. Controlling infection spread from excreta. *Nursing Standard* 1994, **8**(33):29–31.

MacGinley K. Nursing care of the patient with altered body image. *British Journal of Nursing* 1994, **3**(22):1098–1102.

Moppett S. Which way is up for a suppository? *Nursing Times* 2000, **96**(19):NTPlus 12–13.

Naylor J, Mulley G. Commodes: inconvenient conveniences. *British Medical Journal* 1993, **307**:1258–1260.

Parker LJ. Urinary catheter management: minimizing the risk of infection. *British Journal of Nursing* 1999, **8**(9):563–569.

Pellowe C. Prevention of infections from short-term indwelling catheters. *Nursing Times* 2001, **97**(14):34–35.

Scholtes S. Management of clot retention following urological surgery. *Nursing Times* 2002, **98**(28):NT Plus 48–50.

Stewart E. Urinary catheter: selection, maintenance and nursing care. *British Journal of Nursing* 1998, **7**(19):1152–1161.

Smith CE. Assessing bowel sounds: more than just listening. *Nursing* 1988, **18**(2):42–43.

Wells M. Urinalysis. *Professional Nurse Study Supplement* 1997, **13**(2):11–13.

Winn C. Basing catheter care on research principles. *Nursing Standard* 1996, **10**(18):38–40.

Wolf ZR. Bowel management: nursing's hidden work. *Nursing Times* 1996, **92**(21):26–28.

Notes

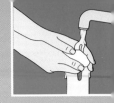

9

Prevention of cross infection

Preparation

Patient

- The hands should be washed before and after all patient contact PFP1 .

Equipment/Environment

- A sink with elbow- or foot-operated mixer taps is best.
- Liquid soap or antiseptic detergent hand-washing solution PFP2 .
- Disposable paper hand towels.
- Foot-operated waste bins.

Nurse

- Remove any rings, jewellery and wristwatches PFP3 .
- Any cuts or abrasions on the hands should be covered by a waterproof, occlusive dressing.

Procedure

1. Adjust the taps so that the temperature is comfortable and the water flow is steady and does not result in splashing the surrounding area. Wet the hands.
2. Apply sufficient soap or antiseptic detergent solution to create a good lather.
3. Rub the hands briskly together, making sure that the thumbs, fingernails, fingertips, palms, backs of the hands and the wrists are thoroughly washed PFP4 .
4. Scrubbing the skin is not recommended as it causes microabrasions. Only if the fingernails are visibly dirty should a nailbrush be used.
5. Continue to wash the hands for at least 10–15 seconds, then rinse thoroughly until all traces of soap/antiseptic detergent are removed PFP5 .
6. Turn off the taps with your foot or elbow and allow the water to run off your hands by holding them with the fingers pointing upwards. If the taps are not elbow- or foot-operated, leave the water running until after drying your hands and then use a paper towel to turn off the taps.
7. Dry your hands using disposable paper towels, working from your fingertips towards the wrists. Thorough drying is essential to minimise the growth of micro-organisms and to prevent the hands becoming sore.
8. Discard the used paper towels according to local policy PFP6 .

Points for practice

1. Alcohol hand-rub may be used instead of washing when the hands are socially clean. The alcohol must be applied to all areas (see below) and the hands then rubbed vigorously until dry. Alcohol effectively reduces microbial counts in clean hands, but it is ineffective if used on hands contaminated with body fluids or excreta.

2. Bars of soap should never be used in clinical areas as they provide the ideal environment for growth of micro-organisms when left sitting on the sink in a pool of water. Liquid soap is usually sufficient for hand-washing in most situations, but an antiseptic detergent hand-washing solution containing chlorhexidine or iodine may be required before procedures such as urinary catheterisation. The local infection control policy will indicate when this is necessary.

3. Local policy may permit the wearing of a wedding ring. This should be a plain band and loose enough to allow washing and drying underneath it. Wrist watches must not be worn as they prevent washing the wrist area.

4. Several research studies have shown that hand-washing techniques are not always effective. Areas of the hands that are commonly missed are the thumbs, fingernails, fingertips, palms, backs of the hands and the wrists (Figure 9.1).

5. The hand-washing technique should take at least 10–15 seconds, preferably 30 seconds (Gould 1994).

6. In some hospitals, hand towels are considered to be clinical waste and so should be discarded in the yellow clinical waste bag. In others they are deemed to be household waste and so should be discarded in the black non-clinical waste bag.

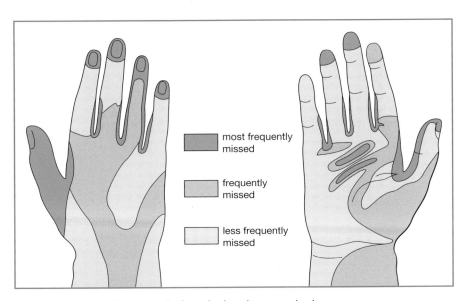

Figure 9.1 Areas often missed when the hands are washed

Preparation

Patient

- Aprons should be worn in all situations where there is direct patient contact or contact with body fluids, bed linen, excreta, clinical waste, etc., or with items that have been in contact with infectious diseases, such as clothes, books, etc.

Equipment/Environment

- Plastic aprons may be available in a variety of colours. In some hospitals, a system exists whereby different-coloured aprons are used for specific purposes, e.g. for serving meals or performing dressings.

Nurse

- The apron should be put on after the hands have been washed.

Procedure

1. Wash and dry your hands thoroughly.
2. Pull the apron over your head; avoid touching your hair and uniform if possible.
3. Tie the apron loosely at the back to avoid it becoming gathered at the waist, so that water splashes will run off easily.
4. If gloves are required (see page 213), put them on after the apron and remove them before the apron is removed at the end of the procedure.
5. To remove the apron, pull at the top and the sides to break the neckband and waist-ties, and fold the apron in on itself to prevent the spread of micro-organisms. Do not allow your hands to touch your uniform.
6. Discard the used apron into the yellow clinical waste bag.
7. Wash and dry your hands thoroughly (see page 210).

Preparation

Patient

- Gloves should be worn whenever patient care involves dealing with blood or other body fluids.
- Gloves may also be required when there is any contact with a patient who has an infection such as hepatitis or methicillin-resistant *Staphylococcus aureus* (MRSA).

Equipment/Environment

- Seamless, single-use latex or vinyl gloves are recommended. These fit either hand and are available in three sizes: large, medium and small.

Nurse

- The use of gloves does not reduce the need for hand-washing. The hands should be washed before and after gloves have been worn **PFP1** .

Procedure

1. It is important to choose the correct size of glove, otherwise dexterity will be severely impaired.
2. If the gloves are required for a 'clean' procedure, such as blood glucose monitoring, they should be taken from those stored in a clean area where they are protected from dust.
3. When removing gloves, do not touch your wrists or hands with the dirty gloves. Using a gloved hand, pinch up the glove of the other hand at the wrist and pull it off turning it inside out. With the non-gloved hand, slip your fingers into the wrist of the other glove and pull it off, again turning it inside out (Figure 9.2).
4. Used gloves must be discarded in the yellow clinical waste bag.
5. Wash and dry the hands thoroughly **PFP2** .

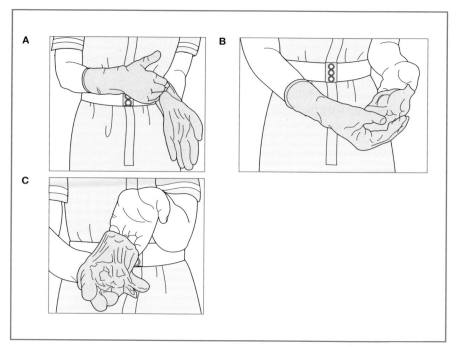

Figure 9.2 Removal of gloves

Points for practice

1. The hands must be washed before and after gloves are worn because the hands sweat within the gloves, creating a warm, moist environment, which encourages micro-organisms to multiply. Also, gloves may not completely protect the hands – they have been shown to develop tiny punctures that go undetected but allow micro-organisms to pass through (Hampton 2002). For information on the use of sterile gloves, see page 224.

2. If an apron is worn, this should be removed after the gloves but before the hands are washed.

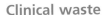

Clinical waste

Any waste generated in healthcare settings that has been in contact with blood or other body fluids is classed as clinical waste and must be incinerated. This includes soiled dressings, swabs, catheters, urine drainage bags, sputum pots, incontinence pads, etc. Used aprons and gloves are also likely to be contaminated by blood or other body fluids and so these should also be classed as clinical waste. All clinical waste must be placed in **yellow plastic bags** for incineration.

Non-clinical waste

Waste generated in hospital that poses no risk to others is classed as non-clinical waste and may be disposed of in the same way as normal household waste. This includes waste such as paper hand towels, newspapers, dead flowers, food packaging, etc. Non-clinical waste should be placed in **black plastic bags** for disposal.

Needles and other sharps

Many procedures in hospitals (and community-care settings) involve the use of needles or other devices capable of puncturing the skin, such as scalpels, lancets, etc. An injury from a needle or other device contaminated with blood or other body fluids poses a high risk to healthcare workers and so special care must be taken when using and disposing of sharps. All sharps must be discarded into special yellow sharps bins, which are rigid, puncture resistant and leakproof (Figure 9.3). They have a special opening which is designed to allow sharps to be dropped easily into the container, but will not allow items to spill out should the container topple over. Sharps bins must not be filled more than three-quarters full, and once closed, they cannot be reopened.

Used needles must never be resheathed and should not be separated from the syringe. If this is unavoidable, a sharps bin with a needle-removing facility on the top should be used so that the needle is not handled. The safe disposal of needles and other sharps is always the responsibility of the person who used them. They should never be left for anyone else to clear away. Where possible, the sharps bin should be taken to the place where the sharps will be used, as this allows immediate disposal after use. If this is not possible, a rigid tray or receiver should be used to contain the sharps until they can be safely tipped, without further handling, into the sharps bin. Never push items into an already full container as this may result in injury.

Linen

Used linen

This refers to all bed linen, clothing, towels, etc., that is used by patients but is not soiled. A plastic apron should be worn when making beds and handling used linen to prevent contact with your uniform. Used linen should be placed in a polythene or fabric linen-bag. These bags must not be overfilled and should be securely fastened to prevent spillage of the contents.

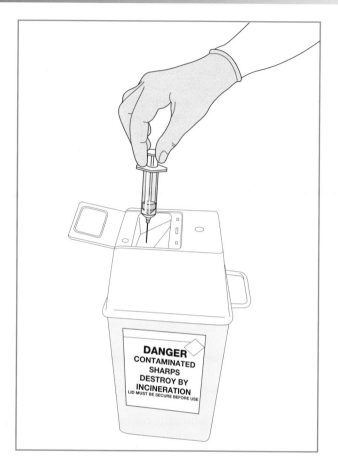

Figure 9.3 Safe disposal of sharps

Soiled or fouled linen

This refers to linen contaminated with blood or other body fluids or excreta. To prevent leakage, this linen should be placed in a plastic bag (the colour of which will vary according to local policy), which should be sealed and then placed in a linen-bag as described above. Personnel wearing protective clothing and gloves will deal with soiled or fouled linen in the laundry.

Infected linen

This refers to linen from patients with infectious conditions such as salmonella, hepatitis, pulmonary tuberculosis or MRSA. This linen must be placed in a plastic bag with a water-soluble seam and then placed in a special fabric linen-bag, which is often red or has red markings on it. In the laundry, the infected linen is not handled by anyone but put straight into a high-temperature (95°C) washing machine in its plastic bag. The water-soluble seam will dissolve during the wash, allowing the linen to be laundered.

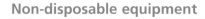

Non-disposable equipment

Although the majority of equipment is now disposable, some items are designed to be reused and this requires sterilisation in the sterile supplies department of the hospital. Such equipment (e.g. surgical instruments, vaginal speculae, etc.) should not be washed after use but placed in a clear plastic bag and returned to the appropriate department for decontamination. There is usually a system whereby all such equipment is placed in a particular bin or bag in the sluice (the colour of this will vary according to local policy), ready for collection.

General equipment

Equipment such as washbowls, commodes, beds and mattresses must be washed thoroughly between patients to avoid cross-infection. These should be cleaned with alcohol wipes or detergent and hot water and dried thoroughly (refer to local policy). All equipment should be stored clean and dry between use. Many hospital wards provide patients with individual washbowls, which are kept in the locker. However, others keep a number of bowls for communal use in the sluice. Abrasive materials should not be used to clean plastic washbowls as this roughens the surface, making it easy for micro-organisms to become trapped. Once washed, bowls should not be stacked one inside the other but upside down in a pyramid to allow the air to circulate freely.

Preparation

Patient

- Explain the procedure, to gain consent and co-operation.
- Ensure comfort and privacy are maintained.

Equipment/Environment

- Sterile swab.
- Plastic specimen bag.
- Laboratory request form.

Nurse

- Wash and dry hands thoroughly.
- Put on apron and gloves.

Procedure

1. Ask/assist the patient to adopt a position that allows access to the appropriate site PFP1.
2. Open the packaging at the handle end and remove the swab, taking care not to contaminate the absorbent tip PFP2.
3. Twist the end of the swab between your finger and thumb to 'roll' the swab so that all areas of the absorbent tip come into contact with the designated area. Avoid touching the surrounding skin PFP3.
4. Open the transport tube and carefully insert the swab. The 'handle' of the swab becomes the stopper or cap of the tube (Figure 9.4).

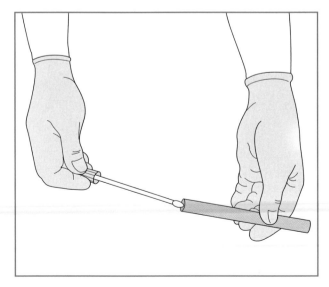

Figure 9.4 Placing the swab in the transport tube

Post procedure

Patient

• Ensure the patient is comfortable.

Equipment/Environment

• Label the specimen container **PFP4** and place it in a plastic specimen bag with the laboratory request form and dispatch to the laboratory or refrigerate as soon as possible.
• Dispose of clinical waste appropriately.

Nurse

• Remove gloves and apron and wash hands.
• Document that the swab has been taken.

Points for practice

1. For MRSA screening, swabs are usually taken from the nose, throat, axillae, groin, perineum and any wounds. A specimen of urine will also be taken if the patient is catheterised (see page 178).

2. The swab may come packed inside its transport tube or it may be packed separately.

3. If the swab is being taken when performing an aseptic dressing technique, this should be done before cleaning/irrigating the wound. If there is no exudate, the tip of the swab may be moistened with transport medium or 0.9% sodium chloride.

4. The patient's details should include: surname; first name; date of birth; hospital number; ward; date and where the swab was taken from (e.g. axilla).

Bibliography/Suggested reading

Bowell B. Preventing infection and its spread. *Surgical Nurse* 1993, **6**(2):5–12.

British Medical Association. *A code of practice for the safe use and disposal of sharps.* London: BMA; 1990.

Bursey S, Hardy C, Gregson R. Hand washing. *Professional Nurse* 2002, **16**:1417–1419.

Curran E. Protection with plastic aprons. *Nursing Times* 1991, **87**(6):64–68.

Donovan S. Wound infection and wound swabbing. *Professional Nurse* 1998, **13**:757–759.

Gould D, Chamberling A. *Staphylococcus aureus*: a review of the literature. *Journal of Clinical Nursing* 1995, **4**:5–12.

Gould D. Hand decontamination. *Nursing Times* 2002, **98**(46):48–49.

Gould D. Preventing cross infection. *Nursing Times* 2002, **98**(46):50–51.

Hampton S. The appropriate use of gloves to reduce allergies and infection. *British Journal of Nursing* 2002, **11**:1120–1124.

Heenan A. Handwashing solutions (techniques and range of solutions available). *Professional Nurse* 1996, **11**(9):615–618.

Horton R, Parker L. *Informed infection control practice.* Edinburgh: Churchill Livingstone; 1997.

May D, Brewer S. Sharps injury: prevention and management. Nursing Standard 2001, **15**(32):45–53.

O'Connor H. Decontaminating beds and mattresses. *Nursing Times* 2000, **96**(46):NTPlus pp 2–5.

Pratt R, Pellowe C, Loveday H et al. The EPIC project: Developing national evidence-based guidelines for preventing healthcare associated infections. *Journal of Hospital Infection* 2001, **47**(Supplement): S3–S4. Also available at *www.doh.gov.uk/HAI.*

Roberts M. Reservoir bugs: sources of hospital-acquired infection. *Nursing Times* 2001, **97**(46):NTPlus pp 54–55.

Royal College of Nursing. *Guidance on infection control in hospitals.* London: RCN; 1994.

Royal College of Nursing. *Universal precautions.* London: Royal College of Nursing; 1997.

Sanderson P, Weisser S. Recovery of coliforms from the hands of nurses and patients: activities leading to contamination. *Journal of Hospital Infection* 1992, **21**(2):85–95.

Starr S, MacLeod T. Wound swabbing technique. *Nursing Times* 2003, **99**(5):57, 59.

Willis J. Skin care: principles of hand-washing. *Nursing Times* 1995, **91**(44):43–44.

York V. Using protective clothing. *Nursing Times* 2002, **98**(46):52.

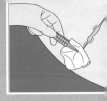

10

Wound assessment

Preparation

Patient

- Explain the procedure, to gain consent and co-operation.
- Assess the wound dressing **PFP1**.
- Check patient comfort, e.g. position, convenience, need for toilet, etc.
- Administer analgesics as appropriate and allow time to take effect.

Equipment/Environment

- Dressing trolley or other suitable surface.
- Dressing pack, syringe (for irrigating the wound), cleansing solution and new dressing according to the care plan/local policy **PFP2**.
- Alcohol hand-rub or handwashing facilities.
- Draw screens around the bed and ensure adequate light. Clear the bed area, close windows, turn off fans, etc.
- Adjust bedclothes to permit easy access to the wound but maintain warmth and dignity.

Nurse

- Consult the care plan to determine the type of dressing required, frequency of change, etc.
- Make sure hair is tied back securely.
- Wash and dry hands thoroughly.
- An apron should be worn.

Procedure

1. Clean the trolley or other appropriate surface according to local policy **PFP3**.
2. Gather the equipment, check the sterility and expiry date of all equipment and solutions, and place on the bottom of the trolley.
3. If scissors are needed to cut non-sterile tape, wash your own scissors, dry them thoroughly and then clean them with an alcohol-impregnated swab. If sterile scissors are needed, these may be included in the dressing pack or packed separately.
4. Take the trolley to the bed area **PFP4**. Adjust the bed to a convenient height to avoid stooping.
5. Remove the dressing pack from its outer packaging, place it on the trolley/surface and taking care to maintain sterility, ease open the pack to reveal the contents.
6. Remove the yellow waste bag and place it to one side.
7. Using your fingertips and touching the edges of the paper only, open the pack and lay it flat to create a sterile field (Figure 10.1).
8. Touching the edges only, move the glove pack to the edge of the sterile field.
9. Pour the cleansing solution and open the dressing, syringe, etc., onto the sterile field. If non-sterile tape is to be used, cut/tear it now and attach it to the trolley in a convenient place for use later.

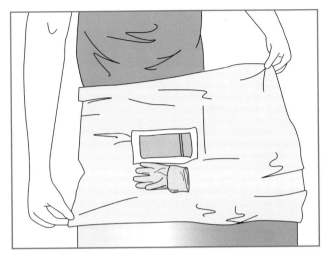

Figure 10.1 Opening the dressing pack

10. Adjust any remaining bedclothes to expose the wound, then loosen the existing dressing but do not remove it **PFP5**.
11. Wash your hands or use alcohol hand-rub. Ensure your hands are completely dry before proceeding.
12. Open the yellow waste bag and put your hand inside so that the bag acts as a glove. Use this to remove the soiled dressing (Figure 10.2).

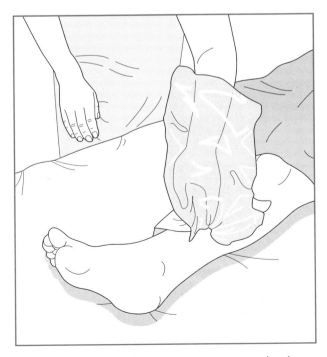

Figure 10.2 Using the clinical waste bag as a glove to remove dressing

13. Inspect the dressing to determine the type and amount of discharge.
14. Turn the bag inside out so that the dressing is contained within it, and using the self-adhesive strip, attach the bag to the side of the trolley.
15. Open the glove pack and taking care not to touch the outside of the gloves, put on the sterile gloves (Figure 10.3).
16. Use a gauze swab dipped in cleansing solution to clean *around* the wound to remove blood, etc. **PFP6**.
17. If the wound itself needs cleaning, use a syringe primed with solution in one hand and a gauze swab on the skin below the wound in the other (Figure 10.4) **PFP7**. Making sure that neither the syringe nor gauze come into contact with the wound, allow the solution to flow into the wound, collecting the solution in the gauze swab held below the wound.
18. Use fresh gauze swabs to dry *around* the wound (not the wound itself), using each swab once only and swabbing away from the wound.
19. Apply the new dressing.

Post procedure

Patient

- When the dressing is secure, replace the bedclothes and assist the patient as necessary into a comfortable position.
- Readjust the bed to a safe height.

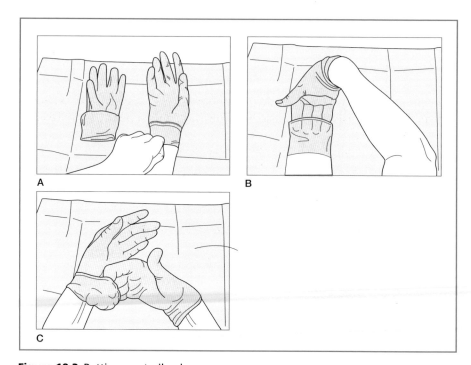

Figure 10.3 Putting on sterile gloves

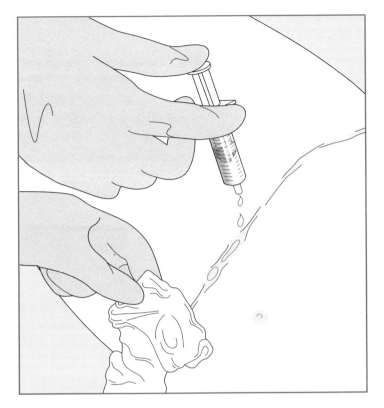

Figure 10.4 Irrigating the wound with saline

Equipment/Environment

- Discard the gloves onto the sterile field. Wrap all used disposable items in the sterile field and place in the waste bag. This should then be tied and placed in the clinical waste.
- Place any sharps, e.g. stitch cutters, in a sharps bin.

Nurse

- Remove apron and wash hands. Return any unused items to the stock cupboard.
- It is not necessary to clean the trolley again unless it has become wet or contaminated with body fluids.
- Document the care given and the condition of the wound. Report any changes or abnormalities.

Points for practice

1. Examine the care plan and the current dressing to determine what type is being used and whether it has been adequate, e.g. whether more padding to absorb exudate is needed.

2. The type of dressing pack will vary according to availability, individual preference and the type of wound.

3. The trolley or surface used must be cleaned thoroughly before use. Local policies may vary, but hot soapy (detergent) water is usually sufficient. It must then be dried thoroughly, to discourage the growth of micro-organisms.

4. In some hospitals, dressings are performed in a clean treatment room rather than at the bedside, to reduce the risk of cross-infection.

5. Leave the existing dressing in place to minimise wound exposure to airborne organisms.

6. Gauze should not be used to clean inside the wound as this has been shown to damage the delicate granulating tissue of a healing wound (Davies 1999). In some hospitals the solution is warmed to prevent cooling and vasoconstriction at the wound site.

7. A syringe (usually 10ml unless the wound is very large) should be used to irrigate gently any wound that needs cleaning. There is a lack of agreement regarding the recommended pressure to use when irrigating the wound (Oliver 1997).

Preparation

Patient

- Explain the procedure, to gain consent and co-operation.
- Check patient comfort, e.g. position, convenience, need for toilet, etc.
- Administer analgesics if appropriate and allow time to take effect **PFP1** .

Equipment/Environment

- Dressing pack containing sterile gloves
- Sterile scissors/stitch cutter and forceps or staple remover as appropriate.
- Alcohol hand-rub or hand-washing facilities.
- Draw screens around the bed and ensure adequate light. Clear bed area, close windows, turn off fan, etc.
- Adjust the bedclothes to permit easy access to the wound but maintain warmth and dignity.

Nurse

- Consult the care plan to determine when the sutures/staples are due for removal, the dressing type, etc.
- Make sure hair is tied back securely.
- Wash and dry hands thoroughly. An apron should be worn.

Procedure

1. Follow the procedure for the aseptic dressing technique to step 9 (see page 222).
2. Taking care to maintain sterility, open the stitch cutter and forceps or staple remover onto the sterile field.
3. Adjust any remaining bedclothes to expose the wound, then loosen the existing dressing but do not remove it.
4. Wash your hands or use alcohol hand rub. Make sure that your hands are completely dry before proceeding.
5. Open the sterile waste bag and put your hand inside so that the bag acts as a glove (see Figure 10.2). Use this to remove and inspect the old dressing.
6. Turn the bag inside out so that the dressing is contained within it, and using the adhesive strip, attach the bag to the side of the trolley.
7. Taking care not to touch the outside of the gloves, put on the sterile gloves (see Figure 10.3).
8. Inspect the wound for signs of healing. If the wound looks inflamed or there is any exudate (pus) present, advice should be sought from an experienced nurse. It may be necessary to remove just one or two sutures/staples to allow the pus to drain.
9. Do not clean the wound before removing the sutures/staples, as cleansing solution may seep into the holes made by the sutures/staples when removed.
10. If the wound is longer than 15cm, remove alternate sutures/staples and check that the wound is fully healed before removing the rest **PFP2** .

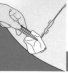

- Individual sutures – if removing individual sutures, use the forceps to lift up the suture. In your other hand, hold the scissors or stitch cutter flat against the skin and slide it under the suture to cut it (Figure 10.5A). In order to prevent infection, the part of the suture that has been lying on the skin must not be drawn underneath the skin and so the place where it is cut is important.
- Continuous suture – when removing a continuous suture, cut the first 'suture' at the end furthest from the knot. Use the forceps to lift the next suture to remove the loose end from under the skin. Cut this suture close to the skin (Figure 10.5B). Repeat this process with all the others, making sure that the part that has been on the skin is not pulled underneath the skin. Never cut both ends of a suture or you will be unable to remove the hidden part underneath the skin.
- Staples – a special instrument is used to remove staples (Figure 10.5C). This should be placed under the centre of the staple and squeezed hard. This bends the staple so that it comes out of the skin easily and does not have to be 'hooked' out. The staple can be steadied, if necessary, by holding it with forceps.

11. Use a gauze swab soaked in cleansing solution to clean and then dry around the wound if necessary (not the wound itself).
12. If there are any small areas where the skin edges are not completely healed together, skin-closure strips may be applied PFP3 .
13. If appropriate, apply the new dressing.

Post procedure

Patient

- Replace the bedclothes and assist the patient as necessary into a comfortable position.
- Readjust the bed to a safe height.

Equipment/Environment

- Wrap all used disposable items in the sterile field and place in the waste bag, which should then be tied and placed in the clinical waste.
- Place any sharps, e.g. stitch cutters, in a sharps bin.

Nurse

- Remove apron and wash hands. Return any unused items to the stock cupboard.
- It is not necessary to clean the trolley again unless it has become wet or contaminated with body fluids.
- Document the care given and the condition of the wound. Report any changes or abnormalities.

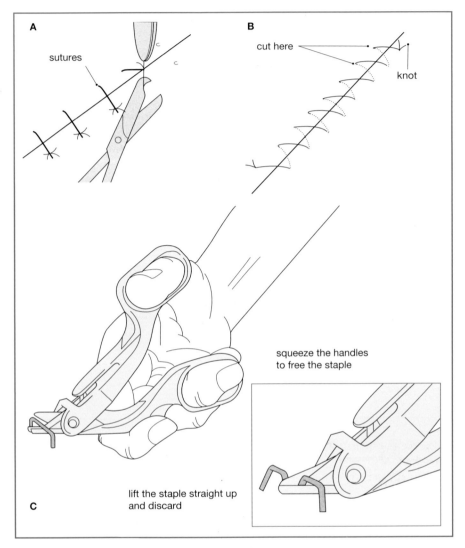

Figure 10.5 A = Suture removal.
B = Removal of a continuous suture.
C = Removal of staples

Points for practice

1. The removal of sutures or staples should not be painful, although the patient may anticipate pain or discomfort. Explanation and careful positioning may alleviate this.

2. If the wound is longer than 15cm or if the incision is in a place where there may be a strain on the skin and underlying tissues, it is better to remove alternate sutures/staples, starting with the second one along. This allows you to check that the wound does not begin to gape at any point before the rest are removed. If this does happen, the remaining sutures/staples may be left until the following day and reassessed. In some instances the number of sutures/staples removed needs to be documented.

3. Skin-closure strips are used to pull the edges of the wound together to promote healing. Attach the strip to the skin on one side of the wound and making sure that the skin edges are aligned without creating excessive tension, lay it over the wound and attach it to the skin on the other side. The next and any subsequent strips should be attached first to alternate sides of the wound (Figure 10.6). This is designed to apply even pressure to the wound edges.

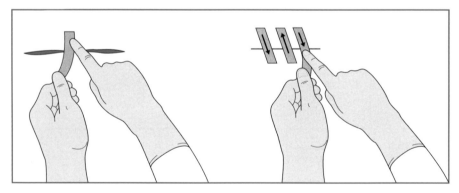

Figure 10.6 Applying skin-closure strips

Principles

Open system

- This refers to a hollow tube or corrugated piece of rubber or plastic that is situated in the wound to promote drainage into the dressing (Figure 10.7). If there is a large amount of drainage, the end of the drain may be inserted into a stoma bag (see page 203). This is designed to keep the wound area free from drainage and thus reduce the risk of infection.

Closed system

- This refers to a system whereby the drain is attached to tubing and a bag for the collection of drainage. This means that the system is 'closed' and thus the risk of infection is greatly reduced. Many closed systems incorporate a vacuum to encourage drainage (Figure 10.8).
- The bag or bottle should be supported by attachment to the bed or patient's clothing to prevent pulling and accidental dislodgement of the drain.
- Asepsis must be maintained when changing the bag or bottle (see page 233).

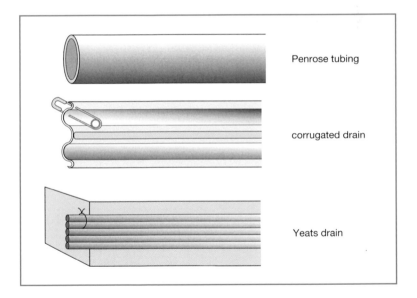

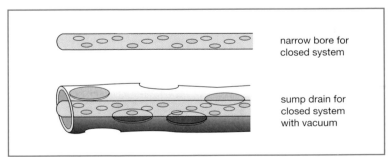

Figure 10.7 Types of drain available

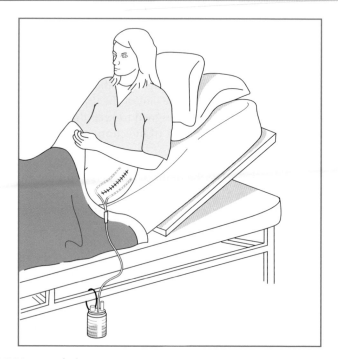

Figure 10.8 Vacuum drainage system

Preparation

Patient

- Explain the procedure, to gain consent and co-operation.

Equipment/Environment

- New vacuum drainage bottle (check that a vacuum is present) **PFP1**.
- Yellow clinical waste bag.

Nurse

- Wash and dry hands thoroughly.
- Put on apron and gloves.
- If there is a danger of splashing, goggles should be worn **PFP2**.

Procedure

1. Detach the drainage bottle from the bed, taking care not to let the bottle slip or the drainage tube may be pulled out.
2. With the clamps that are provided as part of the system, clamp off both the drainage tube (above the connection to the bottle) and the bottle.
3. Carefully remove the drainage tube from the 'old' bottle, taking care not to touch the last 2–3cm to keep it sterile.
4. Note the volume of drainage, then discard the bottle with its contents into the clinical waste bag **PFP3**.
5. Push the tubing firmly into the new bottle and release the vacuum clamp. Release the clamp on the drainage tubing.
6. Secure the bottle to the bed or patient's clothing to prevent pulling.

Post procedure

Patient

- Ensure the patient is comfortable and the drain is not pulling.

Equipment/Environment

- Dispose of equipment and clinical waste appropriately.

Nurse

- Remove gloves and apron and wash hands.
- Document the amount and type of drainage.

Points for practice

1. In one type of bottle, the presence of a vacuum is indicated by the small concertina of plastic folds at the top of the bottle. When the vacuum is no longer present, the concertina effect is lost. If only a small amount of drainage is expected, a small concertina bottle may be used. This is squeezed flat to create a vacuum and then the stopper is replaced to maintain the vacuum.

2. If there is a risk of splashing during the bottle change, goggles should be worn. However, nurses who wear spectacles do not need to wear goggles.

3. The used bottle once clamped, should be discarded into the yellow clinical waste bag. It should not be emptied because of the risk of splashing and contact with blood. However, the drainage in a small concertina bottle will need to be emptied into a jug to be measured. The bottle can be detached, emptied and squeezed flat again to re-create the vacuum. Care must be taken to avoid splashing and goggles should be worn.

Preparation

Patient

- Explain the procedure, to gain consent and co-operation.
- Prepare the patient as described on page 222.

Equipment/Environment

As for the aseptic dressing technique using gloves (see page 222) plus:
- Sterile stitch cutter or sterile scissors.
- Sterile forceps.
- Sterile dressing towel.

Nurse

- Wash and dry hands thoroughly.
- Put on apron.

Procedure

1. Prepare the patient, bed area and equipment as described for the aseptic dressing technique (see page 222).
2. If the drain has a vacuum bottle attached, clamp the tubing with the clamp provided, to release the vacuum and prevent suction during removal of the drain **PFP1**. Detach the bottle, note the amount of drainage and discard the bottle into the clinical waste.
3. Put on sterile gloves and clean the site, if necessary, so that the knot of the suture holding the drain in place is visible and accessible **PFP2**. Place the sterile towel under tubing.
4. Lift up the knot of the suture with the sterile forceps, and using the stitch cutter, cut the suture close to the skin, and remove the suture (see page 228).
5. Fold a gauze swab several times to create an absorbent pad and hold this over the site.
6. Warning the patient of a pulling sensation, gently remove the drain onto the sterile towel. Use counter-pressure on the skin with the other hand if resistance is felt **PFP3**.
7. Maintain pressure over the site until bleeding/drainage is minimal. Cover the drain site with a sterile dressing.

Post procedure

Patient

- Ensure the patient is comfortable.

Equipment/Environment

- Dispose of all sharps and other clinical waste appropriately.
- Scissors, if not disposable, should be returned to the sterile supplies department for decontamination.

Nurse

- Remove gloves and apron and wash hands.
- Document the time and date of removal and the amount and type of drainage.

Points for practice

1. Clamping the tubing prevents suction during removal, which may be painful for the patient.

2. If the drain site appears inflamed or purulent, a swab for culture and sensitivity should be taken (see page 218).

3. Check that the entire drain has been removed. If the drain cannot easily be removed, leave it in position and report it to the nurse in charge.

Bibliography/Suggested reading

Bale S, Jones V. *Wound care nursing: a patient-centred approach*. London: Ballière Tindall; 1997.

Briggs M, Wilson S, Fuller A. The principles of aseptic technique in wound care. *Professional Nurse* 1996, **11**(12):805–808.

Davies, C. Cleansing rites and wrongs. *Nursing Times* 1999, **95**(43):71–75.

Dealey C. *The care of wounds: a guide for nurses*, 2nd edn. Oxford, Blackwell Science; 1999.

Fletcher J. Wound cleansing. *Professional Nurse* 1997, **12**:793–796.

Gottrup D. Wound closure techniques. *Journal of Wound Care* 1999, **8**:397–400.

Leaper D. Antiseptics in wound healing. *Nursing Times* 1996, **92**(39):63–68.

Oliver L. Wound cleansing. *Nursing Standard* 1997, **11**(20):47–51.

Trevelyan J. Wound cleansing: principles and practice. *Nursing Times* 1996, **92**(16):46–47.

Notes

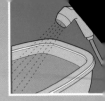

11

Patient hygiene

Preparation

Patient

- Discuss the patient's preference for a bath or a shower.
- Explain the procedure, to gain consent and co-operation.

Equipment/Environment

- Soap/shower gel or antiseptic cleansing agent, according to local policy **PFP1**.
- Flannel/sponge and towels.
- Brush and/or comb.
- Toothbrush, toothpaste and denture pot if appropriate.
- Shampoo (if required).
- Clean clothing.
- Toiletries, make-up, etc., according to individual preference.
- Shower stool or plastic chair.
- Hoist and/or other aids to mobility as required.

Nurse

- Put on plastic apron.

Procedure

1. Check that the bathroom is available and that the bath/shower is clean.
2. Run the bath water.
3. Help the patient to collect together clothes and toiletries.
4. Assist the patient to the bathroom and make sure that access by others is restricted, to ensure privacy **PFP2**.
5. For bathing: use your elbow to check that the bath water is the appropriate temperature for the patient.
6. Assist the patient with undressing, maintaining dignity by covering them with a towel.
7. Observe the condition of the patient's skin, especially at the pressure points (see page 299). Note any signs of inflammation, bruising, discoloration or rash. Note the integrity of the skin and its hydration, whether dry, clammy or sweaty, etc.
8. For bathing: assist the patient to get into the bath. A mechanical hoist is likely to be required for immobile patients **PFP3**.

   For showering: assist the patient to sit on the shower stool or chair and adjust the water flow to the correct temperature **PFP3**.

9. Assist the patient to wash. Encourage patients to do as much as they can themselves.
10. If required, assist the patient to wash their hair, using the flannel as an eye-guard to avoid getting shampoo in the eyes.
11. Assist the patient to get out of the bath or shower, using a mechanical hoist if required. Cover the patient with a towel as soon as possible, to provide warmth and maintain dignity.

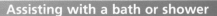

12. Help the patient to dry, apply toiletries as requested, dress in chosen clothing, brush or comb their hair and clean their teeth or dentures as appropriate.
13. Assist the patient to return to bed, chair or day room, using a mechanical hoist if required.

Post procedure

Patient

• Ensure the patient is comfortable.

Equipment/Environment

• Return/replace towels, toiletries, clothing, etc., as appropriate.
• Clean the bath or shower.

Nurse

• Record the procedure in the nursing documentation, noting how much assistance the patient required, the state of the patient's skin and pressure points, and the patient's general condition.
• Report any changes or deterioration

Points for practice

1. Some Trusts require patients to use antiseptic cleansing solution rather than soap, as prophylaxis against methicillin-resistant *Staphylococcus aureus* (MRSA).

2. Ascertain whether the patient wishes to use the toilet before taking them to the bathroom.

3. If leaving patients to wash themselves, make sure they have access to a call bell for assistance.

Preparation

Patient

- Discuss the procedure, to gain co-operation and consent.
- The patient requiring a bed bath will be quite dependent and possibly confused or unconscious.
- Ensure privacy, warmth and dignity.

Equipment/Environment

- Soap or antiseptic cleansing agent **PFP1**.
- Flannel and disposable cloths.
- Two towels.
- Toiletries, make-up, etc., according to individual preference.
- Brush and/or comb.
- Toothbrush and toothpaste, tumbler of water and bowl/receiver.
- Bowl of water (hand hot).
- Clean night clothes.
- Trolley or suitable work surface.
- Linen bag and bags for fouled or infected linen if required.
- Clean bed linen.
- Clinical waste bag.

Nurse

- A plastic apron should be worn.
- Gloves are not necessary unless required by the patient's condition (e.g. MRSA) or if the patient has been incontinent.
- Two nurses may be required for this procedure **PFP2**.

Procedure

1. Assist the patient into a comfortable position. Clear space at bedside for bowl of water and toiletries.
2. Assist the patient to remove any night clothes, ensuring the patient is covered with a sheet or blanket to maintain warmth and dignity.
3. Assist the patient to wash the face, ears and neck. If soap is used, rinse well and dry thoroughly.
4. Wash, rinse and dry the body in a logical order, exposing only the part of the body to be washed. The suggested order is arms, chest, abdomen, genital area, legs, feet and then back **PFP3**; however, this should be discussed with the patient to ascertain any preferences. Change the water as it cools or becomes dirty. If two nurses are present, one should wash and rinse while the other dries the body and applies toiletries as requested, e.g. talc, deodorant or body cream. This reduces the amount of time the body is exposed.
5. As the patient is washed, observe the condition of the skin. Note any signs of inflammation, bruising, discoloration or rash. Note the integrity of the skin and its hydration, e.g. whether dry, clammy or sweaty, etc.

6. Assist the patient to wash, rinse and dry the genital area using a disposable cloth **PFP4** . Remember to wash from the front of the perineal area to the back. In males, ensure that the foreskin is repositioned after washing and drying underneath it. If a urinary catheter is in place, wash carefully around the urethral meatus and catheter tubing, moving away from the meatus, and dry carefully (see page 191). Change the water after washing the genital area.
7. Assist the patient to put on night clothes.
8. Remove any soiled bed linen and remake the bed. This is likely to require a second nurse.
9. Assist the patient to clean teeth or dentures (see page 246). If the patient is going to sit out of bed after the bed bath, it is often easier to clean the teeth when sitting in a chair.
10. Assist the patient to brush or comb hair and to clean and file nails if necessary (see page 254).

Post procedure

Patient

- Ensure the patient is comfortable and has required belongings within reach.

Equipment/Environment

- Wash and dry the bowl (see page 217).
- Rinse the flannel under running water to remove all soap, and allow to dry.
- Discard disposable cloths into the clinical waste.
- Return the linen bag to its collection point.

Nurse

- Remove apron and wash hands.
- Record the procedure in the nursing documentation, noting how much the patient could do without assistance and the condition of the skin, eyes, mouth, etc.

Points for practice

1. Some Trusts require patients to use an antiseptic cleansing solution instead of soap as part of their infection control policy. Patients may prefer not to use soap on their face and, if they have any skin condition, may use an emulsifying ointment in the water instead of soap.

2. A bed bath can be carried out with one nurse, but for severely weak or unconscious patients two nurses are required.

3. The back is left until last so that it can be washed and the clean sheet inserted at the same time, to prevent unnecessary movement for the patient. One nurse can often manage until this point, but will need assistance to roll the patient and make the bed with clean linen.

4. Some nurses prefer to wear gloves when washing the genital area.

Preparation

Patient

- Explain the procedure, to gain consent and co-operation.
- Ask the patient to sit upright if their condition allows

Equipment/Environment

- Pen torch or other suitable light source.
- Tongue depressor.
- Disposable gloves.

Nurse

- Wash and dry hands thoroughly.

Procedure

1. Observe the patient's lips, noting whether they are normal or dry and whether there is any evidence of ulcers, sores, cracks or bleeding.
2. Ascertain whether the patient has any dentures. Note their fit and then ask the patient to remove them. Note the condition of the dentures: whether they are clean, stained, warped or cracked.
3. Place the dentures in water, as they will become warped if left dry for long periods.
4. Put on gloves and using the torch, inspect the patient's teeth, noting any decay, white patches (oral thrush), debris or plaque. Identify any worn or loose teeth.
5. Using the tongue depressor and torch, inspect the inside of the mouth, paying attention to the gums, tongue and mucous membranes **PFP1** . Observe whether they are moist, pink and healthy looking or whether there are any blistered, ulcerated or cracked areas. Note any inflammation, swelling or bleeding of the gums and mucous membranes. Note the presence of any halitosis.
6. While inspecting the mouth, note the consistency and amount of any saliva that is present.
7. Ascertain whether the patient has any difficulty with speech, chewing or swallowing.
8. Discuss the patient's usual oral hygiene measures and assess whether assistance will be required with oral hygiene.

Post procedure

Patient

- Offer the patient water to rinse the mouth.
- Explain any further interventions that might be necessary.
- Ensure the patient is comfortable.

Equipment/Environment

- Clear away equipment.
- Discard gloves into the clinical waste.

Nurse

- Wash and dry hands thoroughly.
- Liaise with medical staff if any medication or referrals are required.
- Document the oral assessment in the nursing records.

Points for practice

1. If the patient is unconscious, two nurses may be required – one to carry out the assessment and one to support the patient's jaw during inspection.

Preparation

Patient

- Explain the procedure, to gain consent and co-operation.
- Ensure privacy.
- Help the patient into a comfortable sitting position. If the patient is unconscious, position them on their side.

Equipment/Environment

- Towel and tissues.
- Toothbrush (preferably soft with a small head).
- Toothpaste/denture cleaning paste.
- Container for dentures if required.
- Beaker of water and bowl or receiver.
- Mouthwash solution (e.g. glycothymoline) if required **PFP1**.
- Cleansing agent (e.g. weak sodium bicarbonate) if required **PFP2**.
- Foam sticks if required.
- Lip lubricant if required.
- Suction equipment if required.
- Clinical waste bag.

Nurse

- Wash and dry hands thoroughly.
- Put on gloves and apron.

Procedure

1. Cover the patient's chest with a towel. If the patient is unconscious, cover the bed/pillow with a waterproof cover and a towel.
2. If applicable, remove the patient's dentures and place them in clean water.
3. Using a toothbrush and small amount of toothpaste, clean the teeth, gums and tongue, taking care not to cause any trauma to the mouth. Small side-to-side or circular strokes are the most effective. Remember to clean both the inner and outer aspects of the teeth **PFP3**.
4. If the patient has a particularly dirty mouth due to tenacious mucus or trapped food, a weak solution of sodium bicarbonate may be used – dip foam sticks into a freshly made solution and gently wipe these around the mouth **PFP4**.
5. Following cleaning, the mouth should be rinsed with water to remove any debris or remaining toothpaste which can have a drying effect on the oral mucosa. The patient should be encouraged to rinse vigorously and then spit the fluid into a bowl. If the patient is unconscious, the mouth should be rinsed by using foam sticks dipped in water. Gentle suction may be used to remove fluid or excess secretions (see page 282).
6. If the patient has dentures, these should be cleaned with a toothbrush and denture-cleaning paste and rinsed thoroughly before giving them back to the

patient. Ordinary toothpaste should not be used as this is too abrasive. Do not dry the dentures as this makes them difficult to insert **PFP5** .

7. If the lips are dry, a thin layer of petroleum jelly or lip balm may be applied.

Post procedure

Patient

- Ensure the patient is comfortable.
- Inspect the mouth (see page 244).

Equipment/Environment

- Rinse the toothbrush and replace the toothbrush and toothpaste in the patient's locker.
- Discard or if required frequently, cover any unused cleaning solution **PFP6** .
- Discard used equipment into the clinical waste.

Nurse

- Remove gloves and apron and wash hands.
- Document any abnormalities or improvements in the patient's oral condition in the nursing records.

Points for practice

1. Some patients may prefer to rinse their mouth with a mouthwash solution after their teeth and mouth have been cleaned. This is very refreshing but the effect is only short-lived and so mouthwash needs to be offered frequently.

2. If sodium bicarbonate solution is required, a weak solution should be prepared by mixing a very small amount (equivalent to 1 teaspoon in 500ml) in a tumbler of water. If the solution is too strong it may damage the oral mucosa.

3. If patients have oral thrush (*Candida albicans*), their dentures should be soaked in a chlorhexidine solution for at least 10 minutes to minimise the risk of re-infection.

4. A toothbrush is always preferable. Foam sticks are not effective in removing plaque from the surface of teeth but they are useful for rinsing or refreshing the mouth.

5. Unconscious patients should not wear their dentures, as these may obstruct the airway. The dentures should be cleaned and stored in water in a labelled denture pot.

6. Any solutions prepared for mouth care must be kept covered between uses and should be discarded and replaced every 24 hours.

Preparation

Patient

- Ascertain the patient's preferences for shaving and incorporate this into the hygiene routine accordingly.
- If possible, the patient should be sitting up.

Equipment/Environment

- Bowl of hot water.
- Flannel/disposable cloth and towel.
- Shaving cream or soap.
- Razor **PFP1** .
- Aftershave/cologne according to individual preference.

Nurse

- Wash and dry hands thoroughly.
- Put on apron.

Procedure

1. Drape a towel across the patient's chest.
2. Ask/assist the patient to wash their face. Inspect the face for any raised areas such as moles or sores.
3. Apply the shaving cream or soap to the face, creating a good lather.
4. Using short strokes of the razor in the direction of the hair growth, shave the face starting with the cheeks and moving down towards the neck **PFP2** . Avoid any raised area such as moles or blemishes.
5. The nurse's free hand should be used to pull the skin taut (Figure 11.1).

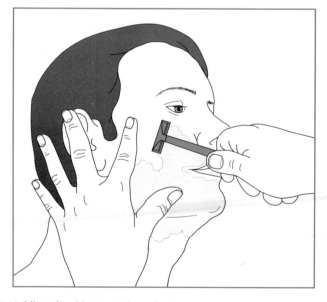

Figure 11.1 Holding the skin taut when shaving

6. Rinse the razor after each stroke.
7. When the entire face and neck have been shaved, rinse the face in clean water and pat dry with a towel.
8. Apply aftershave or cologne if desired.

Post procedure

Patient

- Ensure the patient is comfortable.

Equipment/Environment

- Wash and dry the bowl and replace it in the appropriate storage area (see page 217).
- Rinse the flannel or discard the disposable cloth.
- Discard the razor or dulled razor blades into a sharps bin.
- Replace any personal equipment in the patient's locker.

Nurse

- Remove apron and wash hands.
- Document the procedure, noting how much the patient could do unassisted.

Points for practice

1. Many patients will have their own electric razor and so will not require a wet shave. Communal electric razors should never be used, because of the risk of cross-infection.

2. Patients can often help by making facial movements that tighten the skin being shaved, e.g. filling out cheeks with the tongue.

Preparation

Patient

- Explain the procedure, to gain consent and co-operation.
- Ascertain the patient's preferences regarding hair care.
- Ensure warmth and privacy.

Equipment/Environment

- Plastic sheeting and absorbent pad or towel to protect the bed.
- Shampoo and conditioner if used.
- Comb and/or brush.
- Flannel/disposable cloth and towels
- Two large plastic bowls (one full of hand-hot water, the other empty) **PFP1**
- Clean jug.
- Hairdryer.

Nurse

- An apron should be worn.
- A second nurse may be needed, to support the patient's head and neck.

Procedure

1. Remove the head of the bed.
2. Place the plastic sheeting and the absorbent pad or towel over the pillows, and place the empty bowl on a chair at the top of the bed.
3. Ask/assist the patient to lie on their back at the very top of the bed, with pillows supporting the shoulders and the head positioned over the bowl. Cover the shoulders with a towel (Figure 11.2).
4. Observe the condition of the hair and scalp **PFP2**. Wet the patient's hair by taking warm water from the bowl into the jug and pouring it over the hair, allowing the water to run into the bowl on the chair.

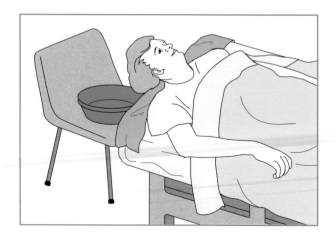

Figure 11.2 Washing the patient's hair in bed

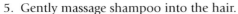

5. Gently massage shampoo into the hair.
6. Rinse the hair with clean water, ensuring that the patient protects their eyes with the flannel or disposable cloth to avoid shampoo getting in. Repeat the process if the patient would like two applications of shampoo and/or conditioner.
7. If conditioner is used, comb it through the hair and leave for 2–3 minutes before rinsing.
8. After the final rinse, wrap the patient's hair in a towel and remove the bowl of water.
9. Assist the patient into a sitting position (if their condition allows) and towel dry the hair.
10. Brush or comb the hair into the desired style, using a hairdryer if one is available.

Post procedure

Patient

- Ensure the patient is comfortable and in a warm environment until the hair is dry.

Equipment/Environment

- Replace the head of the bed and arrange the pillows.
- Dispose of equipment and used towels appropriately.
- Wash and dry bowls and jug, and replace them in the storage area (see page 217).

Nurse

- Remove apron and wash hands.
- Record the procedure in the nursing documentation.

Points for practice

1. Some trusts provide an inflatable hair-washing device that collects the water and so only one bowl is necessary.

2. Before washing the hair, the nurse should assess the condition of the scalp, noting any inflammation, dryness or redness. The condition of the hair should also be noted.

Preparation

Patient

- Explain the procedure, to gain consent and co-operation **PFP1**.
- Assist the patient into a comfortable position, with the head tilted backwards.

Equipment/Environment

- Sterile eye-care pack containing gallipot, gauze swabs and a dressing towel.
- Extra gauze swabs if required.
- Sterile 0.9% sodium chloride (normal saline) solution.
- Clinical waste bag.
- Sterile gloves.

Nurse

- Wash and dry hands thoroughly.
- Put on plastic apron.

Procedure

1. Open the eye-care pack and arrange all equipment on a suitable work surface.
2. Pour the saline solution into the gallipot.
3. Put on the gloves.
4. Ask the patient to close their eyes, and explain which eye is to be cleaned first. Always clean an infected eye last **PFP2**.
5. Lightly moisten a gauze swab with saline, and swab the lower lid from the nose outwards, ensuring that the swab does not rise above the margin of the lid as this could cause corneal damage.
6. Using a new swab each time, repeat step 5 until any discharge or encrustation has been removed.
7. Repeat steps 5 and 6 with the upper lid.
8. Dry the lids by gently wiping with a dry swab.
9. Repeat steps 5–8 with the other eye.

Post procedure

Patient

- Ensure the patient is comfortable.

Equipment/Environment

- Discard equipment into the clinical waste **PFP3**.

Nurse

- Remove gloves and apron and wash hands.
- Record the procedure in the nursing documentation, noting the condition of the eyes.

Points for practice

1. Eye care may be required prior to the administration of eye drops or ointment.

2. If both eyes are infected, two separate eye-care packs should be used.

3. Because of the risk of infection, eye-care packs should not be kept for repeated use. A new pack should be used each time.

Preparation

Patient

- Explain the procedure, to gain consent and co-operation.
- Ascertain usual nail-care habits.
- Carry out this procedure following a bath if possible, as soaking will soften the nails.

Equipment/Environment

- Bowl of warm water.
- Nail clippers or scissors.
- Nail file or emery board.
- Orange stick.
- Hand cream or lotion according to patient preference.
- Towel.

Nurse

- Wash and dry hands thoroughly.
- Put on plastic apron.
- Knowledge of local policy regarding nail care **PFP1**.

Procedure

Fingernails

1. Inspect the hands, fingers and nails, noting any signs of dryness and the condition of the nails and cuticles.
2. If patient has recently had a bath, nail care may proceed. If not, soak the hands in a bowl of warm water for 15 minutes, re-warming the water as necessary.
3. Clean under the fingernails with an orange stick or nail file while the fingers are soaking.
4. Remove the fingers from the bowl and dry them thoroughly.
5. Cut/clip the fingernails level with the top of the finger. The nails can then be smoothed to the shape of the finger with a nail file/emery board.
6. Push the cuticles back gently with an orange stick.
7. Apply cream or lotion as appropriate.

Toenails

1. Inspect the feet and toe nails, noting any dryness, inflammation or cracking. Also note any calluses or ulcerated areas and the colour and temperature of the feet to assess adequacy of circulation.
2. If the patient has recently had a bath, nail care may proceed. If not, soak the feet in a bowl of warm water for 15 minutes, re-warming the water as necessary.
3. Clean and cut the toenails as for fingernails, but cut them straight across and do not file the corners as this may encourage in-growing nails.

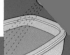

Post procedure

Patient

• Ensure the patient is comfortable.

Equipment/Environment

• Wash and dry the bowl and replace it in the appropriate storage area (see Care of general equipment, page 217).
• Replace any personal equipment in the patient's locker.
• Discard waste into the clinical waste.

Nurse

• Remove apron and wash hands.
• Document the procedure in the nursing records and report any abnormalities, e.g. areas of ulceration or poor peripheral circulation.

Points for practice

1. Check hospital policy on nail care and refer the patient to the chiropodist or medical team, as appropriate, if the patient's condition precludes nurses attending to the nails, e.g. peripheral vascular disease, diabetes or older adults who may have hard or brittle nails.

Preparation

Patient

- Death will have been confirmed **PFP1** .
- Relatives will have been informed and given the opportunity to see the deceased and may participate in the last offices.
- Attention must be paid to the beliefs and wishes of deceased patients and their relatives **PFP2** .
- Screen the bed securely as soon as death occurs.

Equipment/Environment

- Prepare the bed area to ensure sufficient space is available.
- Equipment for bed bath (see page 242).
- Cotton wool, gauze or padding as required.
- Clean sheet and counterpane **PFP3** .
- Tape for securing the sheet.
- Two name bands.
- Two labels from the 'deceased patients book' **PFP4** .
- Property book.
- Shroud.
- Small cotton bandage.
- Receiver (to express bladder).
- Linen bag and clinical waste bag.
- Cadaver bag (if required).

Nurse

- Last offices requires two nurses working together quietly.
- Be familiar with hospital policy regarding last offices.
- An apron should be worn and gloves should be available.

Procedure

1. Take the equipment to the bedside and secure the screens, to prevent accidental opening.
2. Wash the patient. Leave/replace dentures if they fit.
3. Remove any tubes, catheters and infusions unless otherwise indicated, e.g. post-mortem (autopsy) requirements.
4. If leakage is apparent from wounds or orifices, use packing or padding, according to local policy **PFP5** . It may be necessary to express urine from the bladder into the receiver.
5. With the second nurse as a witness, remove all jewellery from the body unless advised otherwise, e.g. Sikhs – leave bracelet (kara). If jewellery is left, this should be covered with adhesive tape or tied in position to prevent loss.
6. Place the shroud on the patient, with the fastening at the back.
7. Place a clean sheet under the patient, leaving enough sheet to fold over the head and feet **PFP6** . Use the bandage to tie the feet together.
8. Place one label on the chest attached to the shroud with adhesive tape.

9. Place one name band on the wrist and the other on the ankle or according to local policy.
10. Wrap the body in the sheet and secure with tape.
11. Place the other label on the chest.
12. If there is a risk of infection, the body may be placed in a cadaver bag. The bag is labelled 'Danger of Infection' plus the name of the infection.
13. Complete the property form. Both nurses must document and sign for any valuables. Any valuables left on the body should also be noted on the death form.

Post procedure

Patient

- Pack the patient's belongings.
- Store property according to local policy, e.g. in the bereavement office.
- Contact porters or mortuary technicians to remove the body.

Equipment/Environment

- Clear away equipment and dispose of clinical waste safely.
- Leave the area tidy, ready for cleaning/disinfecting.
- Flowers, if present, may be left on the bedside locker.
- Ensure that the remaining patients' bed areas are screened when the body is removed, and a calm and quiet approach is adopted.

Nurse

- Remove gloves and apron and wash hands.
- Complete the care plan and other documentation according to local policy.

Points for practice

1. After death, the body is usually left for an hour before last offices are commenced, during which time a doctor or senior nurse will have certified the death. A pillow may be used to support the jaw, to prevent the mouth falling open, and the eyes closed with wet gauze swabs if necessary. The limbs should be straightened if necessary.

2. Religious/cultural preferences must be ascertained prior to last offices, e.g. who can touch the body, non-removal of religious objects or jewellery, etc.

3. If the patient is to be seen by the family after last offices, a coloured counterpane makes the bed look less clinical.

4. The labels used to identify the body are found in the 'deceased patients' or 'death notice' book and must be completed before being torn out, to ensure that all copies are completed at the same time. In some Trusts, the labels are provided with other items (e.g. shroud) in a 'last offices' pack.

5. It is important to prevent leakage from the body, as this is unpleasant and potentially dangerous for porters and mortuary technicians. Refer to local policy regarding packing the body to prevent leakage. This should not be performed if a post-mortem examination (autopsy) is required.

6. When rolling the patient to put in the clean sheet, a deep sigh may be heard. This is due to air being forced out of the lungs.

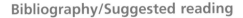

Bibliography/Suggested reading

Baxter C. Caring for patients' hair. *Community Outlook* 1992, **2**(9):29–31.

Barber T. Respect. *Nursing Times* 2001, **97**(47):225.

Buglass A. Oral hygiene. *British Journal of Nursing* 1995, **4**(9):516–519.

Clay M. Oral health in older people. *Nursing Older People* 2000, **12**(7):21–25.

Docherty B. Care of the dying patient. *Professional Nurse* 2000, **15**(12):752.

Glen S, Townley S. Privacy: a key nursing concept. *British Journal of Nursing* 1995, **4**(2):69–72.

Jones CV. The importance of oral hygiene in nutritional support. *British Journal of Nursing* 1998, **7**(2):74, 76–78, 80–82.

Lawler J. *Behind the screens: nursing, somology and the problem of the body*. Melbourne: Churchill Livingstone; 1991.

McGee P. Nursing with dignity. *Nursing Times* 2002, **98**(9):33–35. (This is the first in a series of nine articles designed to help nurses meet the needs of all patients in a multicultural society. The other articles are published in the following eight issues.)

Nyatanga B. Cultural issues in palliative care. *International Journal of Palliative Care* 1997, **3**(4):203–208.

Paterson H. Oral health in long-term care settings. *Nursing Older People* 2000, **12**(7):14–17.

Rader J, Lavelle M, Hoeffer B, McKenzie D. Maintaining cleanliness: an individualised approach. *Journal of Gerontological Nursing* 1996, **22**(3):32–38.

Simmons M. Pre-operative skin preparation. *Professional Nurse* 1998, **13**(7):446–447.

Speck P. Care after death (importance of last offices). *Nursing Times* 1992, **88**(6):20.

Whiting L. Maintaining patients' personal hygiene. *Professional Nurse* 1999, **14**(5):338–340.

Xavier G. The importance of mouth care in preventing infection. *Nursing Standard* 2000, **14**(18):47–51.

Notes

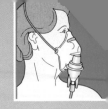

12

Respiratory care

Preparation

Patient

- The patient should be relaxed and resting, or recent activity should be noted.
- Do not inform the patient when you will be assessing breathing PFP1.

Equipment/Environment

- Watch with a second hand.

Nurse

- The hands should be clean.

Procedure

1. Observe the movement of the chest wall and count the respirations for 60 seconds PFP2.
2. Observe the rhythm and depth of respirations.
3. Observe the patient's colour for signs of cyanosis PFP3.
4. Observe for symmetry of chest movement and whether accessory muscles are being used.
5. Observe for the following:
   - Difficulty in breathing.
   - Pain on breathing and its location.
   - Noisy respiration – whether there is any wheeze or stridor.
   - Cough – whether dry or productive.
   - Sputum – amount, colour and consistency (see page 279).

Post procedure

Patient

- Ensure the patient is comfortable. A patient with breathing difficulties may be most comfortable sitting upright (see page 264).

Nurse

- Record the respiratory observations and report any abnormalities.
- Adjust the frequency of observations as necessary.

Points for practice

1. A more accurate observation is obtained if the patient is unaware that their respirations are being counted. Many nurses achieve this by pretending to be feeling the radial pulse when in fact observing the movement of the chest wall (Figure 12.1).

2. If breathing is very shallow and difficult to observe, lightly rest your hand on the patient's chest or abdomen to feel movement. The normal rate for an adult is 12–20 breaths per minute.

3. Cyanosis is a blue discoloration of the skin and mucous membranes and is most noticeable around the lips, ear lobes, mouth and fingertips. In dark-skinned patients, signs of poor perfusion or cyanosis may be detected if the area around the lips or nail beds is dusky in colour.

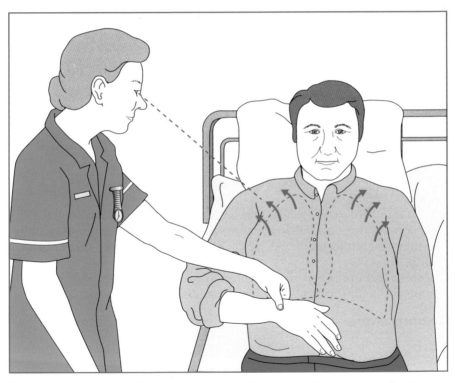

Figure 12.1 Monitoring the respiration rate while apparently counting the pulse

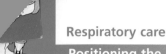

Preparation

Patient

- Explain the procedure, to gain consent and co-operation.
- The patient may be anxious because of the difficulty in breathing.

Equipment/Environment

- Bed with adjustable backrest or electric raising mechanism.
- Four or five pillows.
- Bed table with brakes.
- Firm, supporting armchair.
- A hoist or sliding aid may be needed if the patient is unable to move up the bed unaided.

Nurse

- Two nurses may be needed.
- An apron should be worn if assisting the patient to move.

Procedure

1. Explain to the patient exactly what is planned so that movement is reduced to a minimum.
2. Ask/assist the patient to sit forward. A second nurse may be needed to support the patient while the backrest is adjusted and the pillows are arranged **PFP1**.
3. Adjust the backrest or raise the head of the bed.
4. Arrange the pillows so that the patient feels supported. This will vary according to patient preference but you should ensure that the lumbar region is supported **PFP2**.
5. If the foot of the bed can be raised slightly, this may help to prevent the patient slipping down.
6. For a short period, the patient may get relief by leaning forward with the forearms resting on a pillow on a bed table (Figure 12.2). This may be more comfortable sitting on the side of the bed with the feet supported, or in a chair.
7. If able to get out of bed, the breathless patient is often most comfortable sitting in an armchair, and many prefer to sleep in this position.

Post procedure

Patient

- Observe for changes in respiratory pattern, cough, colour, etc. (see page 262).
- Ensure drink, call bell, etc., are close to hand.

Equipment/Environment

- If sitting for long periods, a pressure-relieving mattress or cushion may be needed to prevent pressure ulcers **PFP3**.

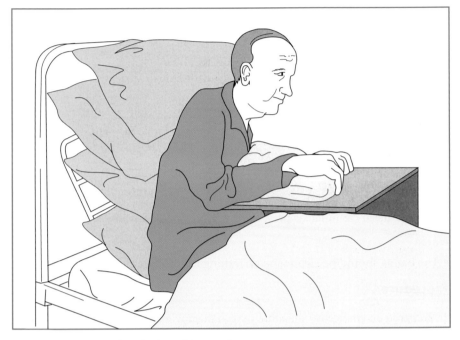

Figure 12.2 Positioning the breathless patient

Nurse

• Document the care given and report any change in condition.

Points for practice

1. When positioning the breathless patient, the aim is to maximise respiratory functioning while reducing physical effort, therefore the patient must be comfortable and well-supported.

2. Ensure the pillows are supporting the small of the back so that the patient does not sink into them and thus restrict chest movement.

3. Regular re-positioning is necessary to prevent pressure ulcers.

Face masks and nasal cannulae

Preparation

Patient

- Explain the procedure, to gain co-operation and consent.
- Prepare the patient preoperatively if oxygen therapy is planned postoperatively.
- Patients and visitors must be made aware of the dangers of smoking when oxygen is being used **PFP1**.

Equipment/Environment

- Oxygen cylinder (if piped oxygen is not available) **PFP2**.
- Oxygen tubing **PFP3**.
- Prescription chart **PFP4**.
- Mask or nasal cannulae as prescribed **PFP5**.

Nurse

- The hands should be clean when handling oxygen equipment.

Procedure

1. Except in an emergency situation, oxygen therapy must be prescribed by a doctor.
2. Turn on the oxygen flow meter and set the flow rate (Figure 12.3B) **PFP6**.
3. Place the mask over the patient's nose and mouth with the elastic strap over the ears to the back of the head. Adjust the length of the strap to ensure the mask fits securely (Figure 12.3A).
4. If using nasal cannulae, place 2cm of tubing into the nostrils; the other tubes go over the ears and either under the chin or behind the head (Figure 12.3C).

Post procedure

Patient

- Observe the patient's colour/perfusion and respiratory pattern.
- Offer drinks or mouth care **PFP7**.

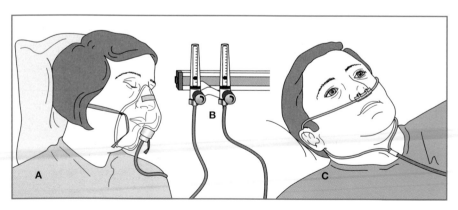

Figure 12.3 A = 'Hudson'-type oxygen mask.
B = Oxygen flow meter.
C = Nasal cannulae

Equipment/Environment

- Tubing and masks may be reused several times for the same patient and should be disposed of in the clinical waste when no longer required.
- If using an oxygen cylinder, ensure that a replacement cylinder is available when the volume indicator gauge shows a quarter full.

Nurse

- Monitor respiratory pattern and rate.
- Document oxygen therapy.

Points for practice

1. Oxygen is highly inflammable.

2. An oxygen cylinder has a black base with white shoulders and has 'oxygen' written on it (Figure 12.4).

3. Oxygen tubing may come in prepacked lengths as a continuous roll with a 'bubble' (widened portion) at regular intervals. Cut through the centre of the bubble and then further trim as necessary to ensure a secure fit onto the flow meter and mask. The length should allow freedom of movement for the patient but not be so long that it may become kinked or touch the floor.

4. Oxygen therapy must be prescribed by a doctor, except in emergency situations.

5. If a percentage of oxygen has been prescribed, a special mask that incorporates a Venturi system is used (Figure 12.5). These are colour coded and specify the flow of oxygen required to deliver 24%, 28%, 35%, 40% and 60% oxygen.

   A Hudson mask is used to deliver a high concentration of oxygen, i.e. greater than 60%.

   If nasal cannulae are used, the flow rate of the oxygen must not exceed 4L/min or it will damage the nasal mucosa.

6. The centre of the ball in the flow meter must sit at the level of the flow rate prescribed.

7. Oxygen therapy dries the mucous membranes of the mouth. Frequent drinks should be taken or frequent mouth care provided if the oxygen is not being humidified. Humidification should always be considered if oxygen therapy is required for prolonged periods (see page 269).

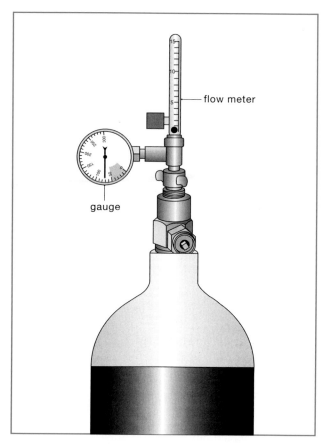

Figure 12.4 Oxygen cylinder

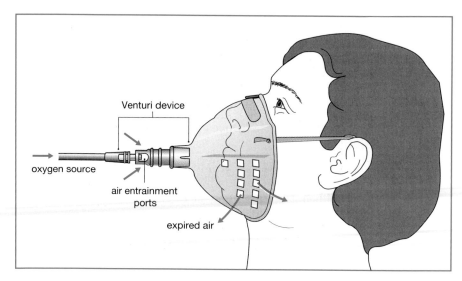

Figure 12.5 Mask with Venturi system

Preparation

Patient
- Explain the procedure, to gain consent and co-operation.

Equipment/Environment
- Oxygen cylinder (if piped oxygen is not available).
- Large-bore 'elephant' tubing.
- Humidifier and water reservoir.

Nurse
- The hands should be clean and the principles of asepsis maintained when handling the water reservoir of the humidifier.

Procedure

1. Check the prescription regarding the percentage of oxygen to be administered **PFP1**.
2. Connect the humidifier to the oxygen flow meter according to the manufacturer's instructions **PFP2**.
3. Connect the wide-bore tubing to the mask and set the flow meter to the flow required to achieve the prescribed percentage of oxygen **PFP3**.
4. A fine mist should appear in the mask. Ask/assist the patient to put on the mask and adjust the retaining strap to prevent pressure on the ears. The nose part of the mask may need to be adjusted to prevent mist going into the eyes (Figure 12.6).

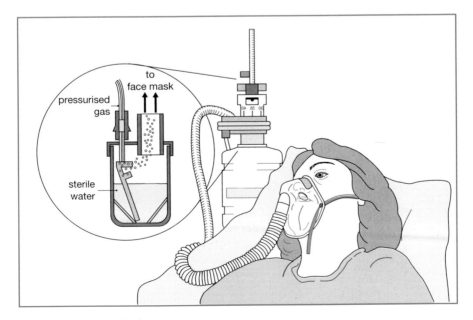

Figure 12.6 Humidified oxygen

Post procedure

Patient

- Ensure the patient is comfortable.
- The humidified oxygen may encourage the patient to cough so a sputum pot and tissues should be provided.

Equipment/Environment

- If using an oxygen cylinder, monitor the amount remaining and order a replacement when it is down to quarter full.
- Empty water from the wide-bore tubing regularly **PFP4**.
- The water reservoir should be replaced when empty.

Nurse

- Document humidified oxygen therapy in the nursing records.

Points for practice

1. Except in an emergency situation, all oxygen therapy must be prescribed by a doctor.

2. Connection will vary according to the type of humidifier. Usually it is achieved by removing the connector at the base of the flow meter, attaching the humidifier by screwing it into position.

3. It is important that the flow is set at the rate indicated to achieve the prescribed percentage. This is usually indicated on the top of the humidifier where it attaches to the flow meter. There may also be a valve adjustment which should be turned to the correct setting.

4. Water that collects in the wide-bore tubing should be emptied by disconnecting the tubing from the humidifier, emptying the water into a bowl or receiver and then reconnecting the tubing. The bowl should then be emptied and kept dry when not in use.

Preparation

Patient

- Explain the procedure, to gain consent and co-operation.
- The patient should be in a comfortable position, sitting upright.

Equipment/Environment

- Air cylinder (if piped air is not available) **PFP1**.
- Nebuliser and face mask or mouthpiece **PFP2**.
- Nebuliser solution **PFP3**.
- Prescription chart **PFP3**.

Nurse

- The hands should be clean and the principles of asepsis maintained when handling the nebuliser and solution.

Procedure

1. Check the nebuliser solution and the patient's identity with the prescription (page 124).
2. Unscrew the base of the nebuliser and add the solution (this is usually in a plastic ampoule that is squeezed to expel the liquid), then screw together again (Figure 12.7A).
3. Make sure the mouthpiece or face mask is securely attached to the nebuliser.
4. Set the flow meter on the air cylinder to 6L/min. A fine mist should appear in the mask and a hissing sound will be heard.
5. Ask/assist the patient to use the mouthpiece or put on the mask by placing the retaining strap over the ears and back of the head (Figure 12.7B).

Post procedure

Patient

- The patient should remain sitting upright until all the solution has been vaporised. This may take up to 10 minutes.
- The nebuliser is likely to encourage the patient to cough so a sputum pot and tissues should be provided.

Equipment/Environment

- If the mask is to be used again, it should be left clean and dry and stored in a plastic bag on the patient's locker.

Nurse

- Document nebuliser therapy according to local policy.
- A peak flow measurement may be requested before and after the nebuliser (see page 273).

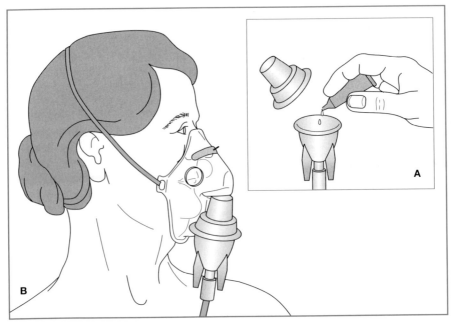

Figure 12.7 A=Adding the nebuliser solution.
B=Nebuliser therapy

Points for practice

1. Nebuliser therapy is administered using air unless high flow oxygen is prescribed. High percentages of oxygen may be dangerous for patients with chronic lung conditions. Check that the cylinder is at least a quarter full.

2. Wherever possible, a mouthpiece is the preferred option as it provides better deposition of the drug into the lungs and reduces side effects (Esmond 2001). If the patient is having nebuliser therapy regularly, the mask or mouthpiece will be kept at the bedside between uses. Nebuliser therapy is usually administered two to four times per day.

3. Drugs to be nebulised (e.g. a bronchodilator) must be prescribed and this must be checked according to local policy (see page 124).

Preparation

Patient

- Explain the procedure, to gain consent and co-operation.
- Ideally the patient should be standing. If the patient's condition does not allow this, they should sit as upright as possible.
- The patient should be rested, as recent exertion may affect the accuracy of the measurement.

Equipment/Environment

- Peak flow meter.
- Disposable mouthpiece.
- Chart to record measurement.

Nurse

- The hands should be clean.

Procedure

1. Attach disposable mouthpiece.
2. Set pointer on the peak flow meter to zero.
3. Instruct the patient to inhale deeply, place their lips around the mouthpiece and holding the meter horizontally, exhale forcibly (Figure 12.8). Make sure that the patient's fingers do not occlude the pointer.
4. Note the measurement.
5. Repeat steps 2–4 twice more **PFP1** .
6. Record the highest of the three measurements (Figure 12.9).

Post procedure

Patient

- Ensure the patient is comfortable.
- Peak flow measurement may be required before and after a nebuliser **PFP2** .

Equipment/Environment

- The disposable mouthpiece may be reused for the same patient. Keep dry and protected from dust.
- Record measurement. Pre- and post-nebuliser recordings should be recorded in different colours to differentiate between them.

Nurse

- Report any abnormality or variation from previous recordings.
- Report any distress caused to the patient by this activity.

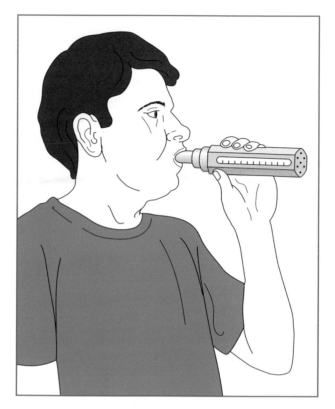

Figure 12.8 Peak flow measurement

Points for practice

1. If the procedure causes the patient distress (e.g. excessive coughing or wheezing), ask the patient to do one recording only. Document this on the chart.

2. If the peak flow rate is to be measured after a nebuliser, this should be done 20 minutes afterwards.

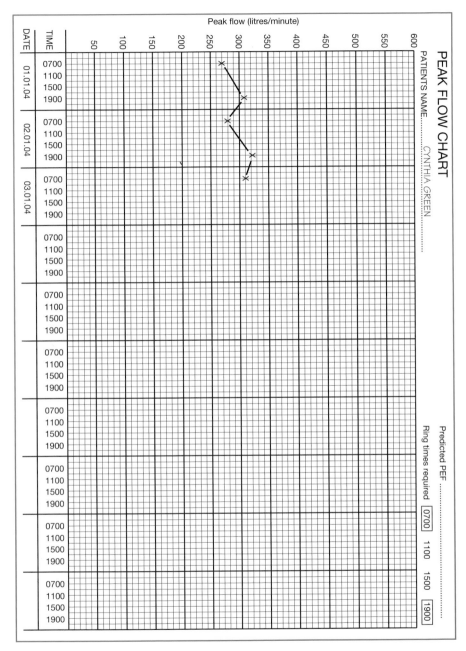

Figure 12.9 Peak flow chart

Preparation

Patient

- Explain procedure to gain co-operation and consent.

Equipment/Environment

- Pulse oximeter **PFP1** .
- Sensor appropriate to patient's size and condition.
- Alcohol-impregnated swabs.

Nurse

- The hands should be clean.

Procedure

1. Assess the patient's peripheral circulation in order to choose an appropriate sensor. The most usual are those that clip onto the patient's finger, although sensors that clip onto the ears or adhesive nasal sensors are available (Figure 12.10).
2. Before applying the sensor, clean the skin with an alcohol-impregnated swab or soap and water and ensure that the skin is clean and dry.
3. If using a finger sensor, remove false nails or nail polish as this could give a false reading **PFP2** . Avoid placing the finger probe on the same arm as a blood pressure cuff as the reading will be inaccurate during inflation of the cuff.

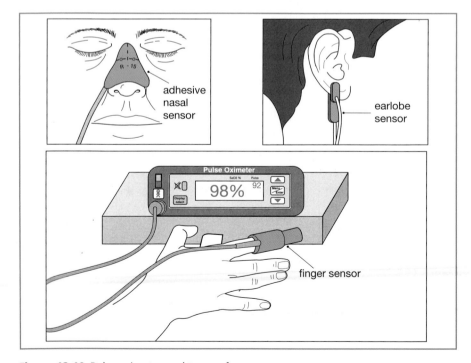

Figure 12.10 Pulse oximeter and types of sensors

4. Attach the sensor according to the manufacturer's instructions then plug the cable into the pulse oximeter and turn on the machine.
5. Observe waveform fluctuations to ensure that the pulse waveform is registering **PFP3**.
6. Set alarm limits on pulse oximeter if not pre-set by manufacturer.
7. If continuous oxygen saturation measurements are required, change the sensor site every 4 hours to prevent pressure damage or irritation from adhesive sensors.
8. If intermittent oxygen saturations are being measured, remove the sensor between readings.

Post procedure

Patient

- Ensure patient is comfortable.
- If using adhesive sensors remove any traces of adhesive with acetone.

Equipment/Environment

- Unplug pulse oximeter and store in equipment storage area.
- Store sensor cable as per manufacturer's recommendations.

Nurse

- Document oxygen saturation measurement in the nursing records, noting whether the patient is receiving oxygen therapy.
- Document the state of the patient's perfusion noting any changes in mental status or colour of the skin.
- Report any change/abnormal findings immediately.

Points for practice

1. The pulse oximeter is used to measure oxygen saturation (SpO_2) levels. The normal level is 95%–99%.

2. Patients with jaundice may give falsely high readings due to high serum bilirubin levels. If the patient has recently had any investigations that involve the injection of radio-opaque dyes, then this may cause spurious readings.

3. Some models of pulse oximeter do not show a pulse waveform, just a digital readout.

Preparation

Patient

- Explain the procedure, to gain consent and co-operation.
- Ensure privacy – the patient may be distressed or embarrassed at having to expectorate.

Equipment/Environment

- Disposable sputum carton with lid.
- Tissues.
- Waste bag.

Nurse

- Gloves should be worn if the patient needs assistance with expectoration, use of tissues, etc.

Procedure

1. Expectoration will be easier if the patient is sitting up, well supported by pillows, or is sitting in an armchair.
2. Encourage the patient to expectorate into the sputum pot rather than swallowing the sputum **PFP1** .
3. Observe the sputum for the following:
   - Quantity.
   - Consistency – whether watery, frothy or tenacious (sticky).
   - Colour: white – mucus; yellow/green – pus (infected); red – fresh blood (haemoptysis).
   - Odour – foul-smelling sputum may indicate a lung abscess.

Post procedure

Patient

- The patient may feel very tired after a bout of coughing.
- A mouthwash or drink should be offered.

Equipment/Environment

- Remove used sputum carton, observe, and then close the lid tightly and discard in the yellow clinical waste bag.
- Provide patient with clean sputum carton

Nurse

- Remove gloves and wash hands.
- Document the amount and nature of the sputum.

Points for practice

1. The assistance of a physiotherapist may be necessary to teach the patient how to breathe deeply and expectorate without strain rather than coughing ineffectively.

Preparation

Patient

- Explain the procedure and the number of specimens required (PFP1).

Equipment/Environment

- Universal specimen pot.
- Plastic specimen bag and laboratory request form.
- Drinking water and mouthwash.
- Tissues.

Nurse

- Gloves should be worn if the patient needs assistance with expectoration, use of tissues, etc.

Procedure

1. Ask the patient to rinse their mouth thoroughly with water (PFP2).
2. Ask/assist the patient to expectorate into the sterile pot (PFP3).
3. Seal the lid and complete the label with the date, patient's full name, hospital number, ward and type of specimen.
4. Place the pot and the laboratory request form in a plastic specimen bag and dispatch to the laboratory or refrigerate straight away.

Post procedure

Patient

- Ensure the patient is comfortable and offer a mouthwash and/or tissues as appropriate.

Equipment/Environment

- Dispose of any waste appropriately.

Nurse

- Document that the specimen has been obtained.
- Note colour, smell and consistency.

Points for practice

1. Three consecutive early-morning specimens may be requested for acid-fast bacilli (tuberculosis) or for cytology (malignant cells).

2. The mouth should be rinsed with water (not mouthwash) before expectoration, to reduce contamination of the specimen.

3. When obtaining the specimen it is important to ensure that it is sputum and not just saliva.

Preparation

Patient

- Explain the procedure, to gain consent and co-operation.
- The patient requiring oral suctioning may be semi-conscious or unconscious **PFP1** .

Equipment/Environment

- Suction machine (if piped suction is not available).
- Suction tubing and oral sucker, e.g. Yankauer sucker (Figure 12.11).
- Sterile distilled water **PFP2** .

Nurse

- The hands must be washed and dried thoroughly.
- An apron and gloves should be worn.
- Goggles will be required if airborne secretions are likely.

Procedure

1. Switch on the suction machine and attach the tubing and oral sucker, ensuring a good fit to prevent loss of suction pressure.
2. If able to co-operate, ask the patient to open their mouth.
3. The oral sucker may have a hole which when occluded by your thumb, enables suction to be applied. If the oral sucker has no suction-control

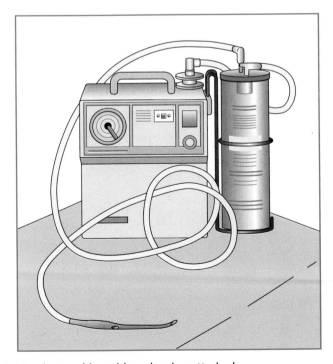

Figure 12.11 Suction machine with oral sucker attached

mechanism, kink the suction tubing so that suction is not applied until required.

4. Gently insert the oral sucker into the mouth, taking care not to make the patient 'gag' by inserting it too far.

5. Apply suction, moving the sucker to all parts of the mouth as necessary.

Post procedure

Patient

- Ensure the patient is comfortable.
- Mouth care may be required following oral suctioning (see page 246).

Equipment/Environment

- Clean the oral sucker and suction tubing by suctioning sterile water through it until all traces of sputum have gone.
- The oral sucker may be used again on the same patient providing it is left clean and covered by a plastic bag between uses. The sucker and tubing should be replaced every 24 hours.
- Replace the cap on the bottle of sterile distilled water.
- If the suction machine has a reusable bottle, this should be emptied at least every 24 hours. Goggles should be worn when emptying it. If it has a disposable sealed container, this does not need to be emptied but sealed and discarded when full or when the patient no longer requires suctioning.

Nurse

- Remove gloves and apron and wash hands.
- Document oral suctioning, noting the amount and appearance of the secretions.

Points for practice

1. Oral suctioning may be required by patients who are able to cough but are too weak to expectorate. It may also be necessary in unconscious patients if there are copious secretions and during cardiopulmonary resuscitation.

2. The sterile distilled water is used to clean the suction tubing after use and must be kept closed to discourage bacterial growth. The bottle must be changed every 24 hours. If poured into a bowl, the bowl must be kept clean and dry when not in use.

Preparation

Patient

- Explain the procedure, to gain consent and co-operation.
- Tracheostomy care is easier if the patient is recumbent or semi-recumbent in bed.

Equipment/Environment

- Sterile dressing pack containing gloves.
- Extra gauze swabs may be needed.
- Dressing trolley or other suitable surface.
- Keyhole dressing according to local policy.
- Two tracheostomy tapes.
- Cleansing solution according to local policy **PFP1** .
- Tracheal dilators **PFP2** .
- Alcohol hand-rub or hand-washing facilities.
- Scissors to cut tapes.

Nurse

- The hands must be washed and dried thoroughly.
- An apron should be worn.
- Two nurses will be needed when changing the tapes (one to hold the tube).

Procedure

1. It is a good idea to perform suction (see page 287) prior to the dressing change, to minimise the risk of coughing and dislodgement of the tube.
2. Prepare the trolley and equipment (see page 222).
3. Raise the bed to a comfortable working height. Remove any humidification/oxygen apparatus from the tracheostomy site, but leave the tapes tied **PFP3,4** .
4. Wash your hands or clean them using alcohol hand-rub.
5. Open the dressing pack, keyhole dressing and cleansing solution, and using the yellow waste bag as a 'glove', remove the old dressing (see page 223).
6. Attach the waste bag to the side of the trolley nearest the patient. Put on the sterile gloves.
7. Use gauze swabs and cleansing solution to clean around the tracheostomy as necessary. Use gauze swabs to gently dry the site.
8. Apply the keyhole dressing (Figure 12.12A).
9. With a second nurse holding the tube in position, cut the tapes, taking care not to cut the pilot tube if it is a cuffed tracheostomy tube, and remove the old tapes.
10. Fold one new tape so that there is a long end (about two-thirds of the length of the tape) and a short end (about one-third of the length of the tape). Thread the folded part through the hole in the flange on the tracheostomy tube (Figure 12.12B) create a loop and thread the rest of the tape through it to secure it. Repeat for the other tape.

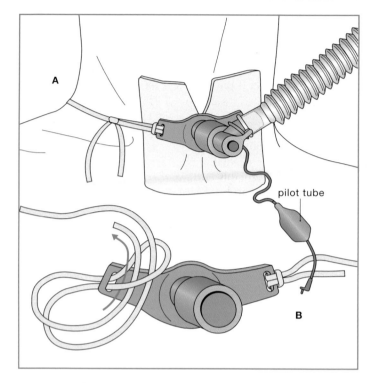

Figure 12.12 A = 'Keyhole' tracheostomy dressing.
B = Threading the tapes through the loop

11. Pass the long end of each tape behind the patient's neck and tie each securely to the short end on the other side. A secure knot, not a bow, must be used to prevent it becoming loose. It should be just possible to slip a finger between the tape and the patient's neck.
12. The long end of the tapes may be threaded through a foam protector before tying, to prevent them cutting into the patient's neck.

Post procedure

Patient

- Replace any humidification/oxygen apparatus.
- Ensure the patient is comfortable and there is no respiratory distress.

Equipment/Environment

- Discard all clinical waste appropriately.

Nurse

- Remove apron and wash hands.
- Document the dressing change, noting the appearance of the tracheostomy site.

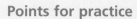

Points for practice

1. The cleansing solution may vary according to local policy but 0.9% sodium chloride is usually sufficient.

2. Tracheal dilators should always be kept by the patient's bedside in case the tracheostomy is dislodged. However, once the tracheostomy is well established, the opening is unlikely to close if the tube is temporarily removed.

3. If the patient is on a ventilator, this must not be disconnected during the dressing change. The second nurse will be able to support the tubing, etc., to facilitate the dressing change.

4. Two nurses are needed to safely change the tracheostomy tapes so that one can hold the tube in position to prevent dislodgement if the patient coughs or moves unexpectedly.

Preparation

Patient

- Explain the procedure, to gain consent and co-operation.
- The patient will have an endotracheal (ET) tube or tracheostomy.

Equipment/Environment

- Suction machine (if piped suction is not available).
- Suction tubing.
- Suction catheters with suction-control mechanism.
- Sterile distilled water **PFP1**.
- Supply of single sterile gloves **PFP2**.
- Yellow clinical waste bag/bin.

Nurse

- Wash and dry hands thoroughly.
- Wear a non-sterile glove on your non-dominant hand and an apron **PFP2**.
- Goggles **PFP3**.

Procedure

1. Turn on the suction machine and test the suction pressure.
2. Open the suction-control end of a suction catheter but leave it in its packet. Attach the end to the suction tubing, ensuring a good fit so that suction pressure is not lost.
3. Place the tubing and suction catheter (still in its packet) in a convenient position ready for use.
4. Open a sterile glove and put it on your dominant hand.
5. With your non-dominant hand, remove any humidifying/oxygen apparatus from the ET tube/tracheostomy **PFP4**.
6. With the same hand, pick up the suction tubing and carefully pull the suction catheter out of its packet.
7. As the suction catheter emerges, take hold of it in your sterile-gloved hand, about halfway down the catheter. Do not allow the catheter to touch anything.
8. Insert the suction catheter into the ET tube/tracheostomy and, after warning the patient, advance it until it reaches the bifurcation of the right and left main bronchi (Figure 12.13). This will make the patient cough **PFP5**.
9. When the patient coughs, withdraw the suction catheter 1–2 cm and then apply suction by occluding the suction-control apparatus with the thumb of your non-dominant hand **PFP6**.
10. Continue to apply suction and gradually withdraw the catheter, rolling it between your fingers and thumb as you do so.
11. Remove the catheter from the ET tube/tracheostomy and wrap it around the fingers of your sterile-gloved hand. Remove the glove, turning it inside out with the catheter contained within it.
12. Disconnect the catheter from the suction tubing and discard.
13. Repeat as necessary using a new catheter and sterile glove each time **PFP7**.

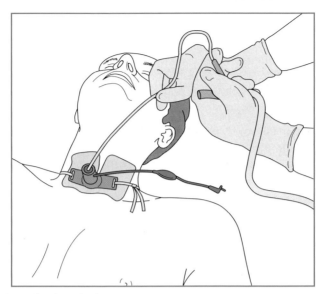

Figure 12.13 Tracheal suctioning

Post procedure

Patient

• Replace any humidification/oxygen apparatus.
• Ensure the patient is comfortable and breathing has returned to its usual rate.

Equipment/Environment

• Clean the suction tubing by suctioning sterile water through it until all traces of sputum have gone. The tubing should be replaced every 24 hours.
• Attach a suction catheter and leave it in its packet ready for next use.
• Replace the cap on the bottle of sterile distilled water.
• If the suction machine has a reusable bottle, this should be emptied at least every 24 hours. Goggles should be worn when emptying it. If it has a disposable sealed container, this does not need to be emptied but sealed and discarded when full or when the patient no longer requires suctioning.

Nurse

• Remove glove and apron and wash hands.
• Document suctioning, noting the amount and appearance of the secretions.

Points for practice

1. The sterile distilled water is used to clean the suction tubing after use and must be kept closed to discourage bacterial growth. The bottle must be changed every 24 hours. If poured into a bowl, the bowl must be kept clean and dry when not in use.

2. A single sterile glove is used with each suction catheter. A non-sterile glove should be worn on your non-dominant hand to prevent contact with tracheal secretions when the suction-control apparatus is occluded with your thumb. If the catheter does not have an integral suction-control mechanism, a 'Y' connector may be inserted to serve the purpose.

3. Some authors recommend that goggles are worn because of the risk of airborne secretions when the patient coughs (Day 2000).

4. If the patient is on a ventilator, the top of the ET tube should be removed at the last minute and replaced immediately after each suctioning. Suction should be performed swiftly, as the patient is unable to breathe unaided. A guide is to hold your own breath as you insert the catheter and aim to complete suctioning by the time you need to breathe again.

5. When the suction catheter touches the tracheal wall, the patient will cough, sometimes violently. Patients find this unpleasant and often distressing, but it is important to induce coughing to prevent stasis of secretions in the lungs. In order to avoid damage to the tracheal wall, the suction catheter should be withdrawn once the bifurcation has been located (McEleney 1998).

6. The suction catheter should be rolled between the fingers as it is withdrawn, to facilitate the removal of secretions and to prevent high pressure being applied to any part of the tracheal wall. The tips of most suction catheters are designed to minimise this.

7. Suctioning should be repeated until the ET tube/tracheostomy is clear of secretions and the breathing sounds clear. However, this may be distressing and so it may be necessary to allow time for the patient to rest during the procedure.

Preparation

Patient

- Explain the procedure, to gain co-operation and consent.
- Explain positioning of the tube and subsequent limitations to mobility.
- Explain the importance of not raising the bottle higher than the patient's chest (see procedure point 9 below).
- Ask/assist the patient to move into the required position – usually sitting forward resting on a table for support.
- Ensure privacy and dignity are maintained throughout.

Equipment/Environment

- Dressing trolley or clean surface.
- Sterile chest drain insertion pack or dressing pack.
- Hypoallergenic adhesive tape.
- Goggles and sterile gown and gloves for doctor.
- Antiseptic skin-cleansing solution according to local policy.
- Local anaesthetic as prescribed.
- Syringes and needles for administration of local anaesthetic.
- Sterile disposable scalpel.
- Suture material (usually silk) for purse-string and retaining suture.
- Sterile chest drain and introducer/trochar.
- Sterile drainage equipment (usually disposable) and sterile water.
- Two tubing clamps **PFP1**.
- Sharps bin.

Nurse

- The nurse's role during chest drain insertion is to observe and support the patient and assist the doctor.
- Record the patient's blood pressure, pulse, respiratory rate and oxygen saturation (if appropriate) as baseline measurements.
- Wash and dry hands thoroughly.
- Put on apron.

Procedure

1. Administer sedative or analgesic (if prescribed) 20 minutes before the procedure.
2. Maintaining the principles of asepsis, assemble the drainage equipment and add the water. Make sure that the tube to be attached to the chest drain tubing is 4–5cm below the water level (Figure 12.14) **PFP2**.
3. Open the sterile pack and add the sterile gown, gloves, syringe, scalpel and suture material.
4. Pour the antiseptic skin-cleansing solution into a gallipot. The doctor will now put on the goggles and sterile gown and gloves.
5. When requested by the doctor, open the sterile needle for attachment to the syringe and hold the ampoule of local anaesthetic for the doctor to check and then draw into the syringe.

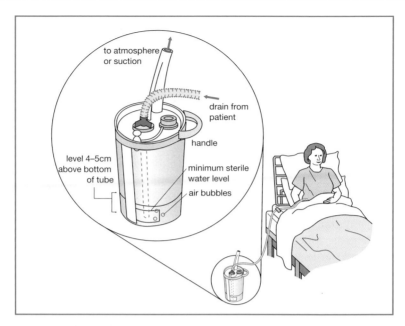

Figure 12.14 Underwater seal chest drain

6. When requested by the doctor, open the packaging of the chest drain and introducer/trochar.
7. During insertion of the chest drain observe the patient for signs of discomfort or respiratory distress.
8. When the chest drain is inserted it should be attached to the drainage bottle immediately. The tubing may be clamped to prevent further lung collapse prior to attachment to the drainage bottle. The drain is then sutured in place and a purse-string suture inserted by the doctor. Remove clamp **PFP3**.
9. The drainage bottle should always be kept below the level of the patient's chest to prevent siphoning of fluid into the pleural space.
10. The drain should be further secured with adhesive tape and the site covered with a dry dressing **PFP4,5**.
11. Check that the drainage system is functioning by observing for swinging movement of water in the drain tubing as the patient breathes. There should be bubbling in the water with respiration in the case of a pneumothorax, and drainage of blood into the bottle in the case of a haemothorax.
12. If suction has been prescribed, the suction tubing is attached to the short tube in the bottle, the one that does not touch the water.

Post procedure

Patient

• Ensure that the patient is comfortable and that the tubing of the chest drain is not pulling or kinked. A chest X-ray will be required to confirm the position of the chest drain.

- Patients should be encouraged to mobilise and sit up where possible. Deep breathing and coughing promote pleural drainage **PFP6** .

Equipment/Environment

- Discard all clinical waste appropriately.
- Discard needles, scalpel and the chest drain introducer into the sharps bin.

Nurse

- Remove apron and wash hands.
- Record the patient's blood pressure, pulse, respiratory rate and oxygen saturation at least 4 hourly.
- Document the chest drain insertion and, if applicable, the amount of suction required **PFP7** .
- Monitor drainage, whether the fluid level is 'swinging' and any air leak.

Points for practice

1. Chest drain tubes should only be clamped if accidental disconnection occurs or when bottles are being changed. Unnecessary clamping of tubes may cause a tension pneumothorax.

2. The end of the long tube in the bottle must be underwater to prevent air being drawn into the lungs during inspiration. It should be no more than 4–5cm beneath the water level as this may make expansion of the lung more difficult.

3. If more than one drain has been inserted, make sure they are clearly labelled (e.g. basal and apical).

4. The tubing can be secured to the patient's clothing by wrapping tape around the tubing and placing a safety pin through the tape. This can prevent the occurrence of kinks in the tubing.

5. To facilitate measurement of the rate of drainage, a piece of tape placed vertically next to the calibrated scale of the bottle can be marked at suitable intervals.

6. Take care that the drainage bottles are not damaged when raising or lowering the bed.

7. Do not turn off the suction without disconnecting the tubing from the chest drain as this has an effect similar to the tube being clamped (see above).

Preparation

Patient

- Explain the procedure, to gain consent and co-operation.
- Instruct the patient to practise deep breathing and holding their breath.
- Ask/assist the patient to adopt an upright position which is comfortable.
- Ensure privacy.

Equipment/Environment

- Dressing trolley or clean work surface.
- Sterile dressing pack containing gloves.
- Extra pair of gloves for the assisting nurse.
- Sterile dressing towel.
- Skin-cleansing solution according to local policy **PFP1**.
- Sterile dressing to cover site.
- Sterile stitch cutter.
- Alcohol hand-rub or hand-washing facilities.
- Large clinical waste bag.
- Sharps bin.

Nurse

- Two nurses are required for this procedure.
- The hands should be washed and dried thoroughly.
- Aprons should be worn.
- Both nurses should wear goggles.

Procedure

1. Administer any prescribed analgesic or sedative **PFP2**.
2. Take the equipment to the bedside and raise the bed to an appropriate height to avoid stooping.
3. Maintaining the principles of asepsis, open the dressing pack and pour the cleansing solution into a gallipot or fluid tray. Open the stitch cutter and dressing onto the sterile field.
4. Loosen the dressing around the drain site but do not remove.
5. Wash your hands or clean them using alcohol hand-rub.
6. Using the waste disposal bag as a 'glove', remove the dressing (see page 223).
7. Put on gloves and clean around the drain site to remove any dried blood or exudate that may impede removal of the drain.
8. Cut the knot at the loose end of the purse-string suture so that the ends are free (Figure 12.15). Cut and remove the suture holding the drain in place (see page 228).
9. Ask the assisting nurse to put on gloves and to tie the purse-string suture loosely **PFP3**.
10. Instruct the patient to take two deep breaths and hold it (this should have been practised beforehand).

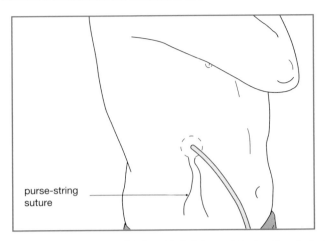

Figure 12.15 Purse-string suture – this is pulled tight and tied as the drain is removed

11. When the patient is holding their breath, the nurse quickly and smoothly removes the chest drain. The assisting nurse pulls the purse-string suture tight and ties it with a double knot. Speed is essential.
12. On completion, instruct the patient to breathe normally.
13. Ask the assisting nurse to disconnect the chest drain tubing and discard it in the clinical waste bag **PFP4** .
14. Clean any fluid or exudate from the drain site and cover it with a dry dressing.

Post procedure

Patient

- Ensure the patient is comfortable **PFP5** .
- Instruct the patient to report any breathlessness/difficulty in breathing.
- The doctor may order a chest X-ray following removal of the chest drain.

Equipment/Environment

- Dispose of all waste and equipment appropriately.
- The chest drain bottle and tubing is usually disposable and can be discarded in the clinical waste. If it is not disposable, it should be returned to the sterile services department according to local policy.

Nurse

- Remove gloves, apron and goggles and wash hands.
- Record chest drain removal in the nursing documentation. Remember to measure and record the final fluid drainage.

Points for practice

1. The skin-cleansing solution used may vary according to local policy but 0.9% sodium chloride is usually sufficient.

2. The doctor may prescribe analgesia or a sedative prior to chest drain removal; this should be given at least 20 minutes before the procedure.

3. If the drain was on suction, this should be disconnected before chest drain removal.

4. If two chest drains are connected to one bottle, clamp each drain close to the patient's chest and disconnect the tubing from the bottle prior to removal.

5. The purse-string suture can be removed after 5 days.

Bibliography/Suggested reading

Assessment of breathing

Baxter C. Observing skin (making an accurate diagnosis in people with dark skin). *Community Outlook* 1993, **3**(1):21–22.

Esmond G. *Respiratory nursing.* Edinburgh, Ballière Tindall, 2001.

Jevon P, Ewens B. Assessment of a breathless patient. *Nursing Standard* 2001, **15**(16):48–50.

Kenward G, Hodgetts T, Castle N. Time to put the R back into TPR. *Nursing Times* 2001, **97**(40):32–33.

Law C. A guide to assessing sputum. *NT Plus* 2000, **96**(24):7–10.

Oxygen therapy

Ashurst S. Oxygen therapy. *British Journal of Nursing* 1995, **4**(9):508–515.

Bambridge AD. An audit of comfort and convenience: comparison of oxygen mask and nasal catheter in the provision of post-operative oxygen therapy. *Professional Nurse* 1993, **8**(8):513, 515–518.

Bateman NT, Leach RM. ABC of oxygen: acute oxygen therapy. *British Medical Journal* 1998, **317**:761, 798–801.

Bell C. Is this what the doctor ordered? Accuracy of oxygen therapy prescribed and delivered in hospital. *Professional Nurse* 1995, **10**(5):297–300.

Esmond G. Nebuliser therapy. *Professional Nurse* 1998, **14**(1):30–43.

Pulse oximetry

Cowan T. Pulse oximeters. *Professional Nurse* 1997, **12**(10):744–750.

Howell M. Pulse oximetry: an audit of nursing and medical staff understanding. *British Journal of Nursing* 2002, **11**(3):191–197.

Sims J. Making sense of pulse oximetry and oxygen dissociation curve. *Nursing Times* 1996, **92**(1):34–35.

Sinex JE. Pulse oximetry: principles and limitations. *American Journal of Emergency Medicine* 1999, **17**(1):59–66.

Woodrow P. Pulse oximetry. *Nursing Standard* 1999, **13**(42):42–46

Chest drains

Avery S. Insertion and management of chest drains. *Nursing Times* 2000, **96**(37): NT Plus pp.3–6.

Godden JR, Hiley C. Managing the patient with a chest drain: a review. *Nursing Standard* 1998, **12**(32):35–39.

Gray E. Pain management for patients with chest drains. *Emergency Nurse* 2000, **8**(1):28–32.

Tooley C. The management and care of chest drains. *Nursing Times* 2002, **98**(26):NTPlus pp. 48, 50.

Tracheostomy

Dat T. Tracheal suctioning: when, why and how. *Nursing Times* 2000, **96**(20):NTPlus pp 13–15.

Harkin H. Tracheostomy management. *Nursing Times* 1998, **94**(21):56–58.

Hooper M. Nursing care of the patient with a tracheostomy. *Nursing Standard* 1996, **10**(34):40–43.

McEleney M. Endotracheal suction. *Professional Nurse* 1998, **13**(6):373–376.

Notes

13

Immobility and associated problems

Employers' responsibilities

The implementation of a number of European Directives in 1992 led to important changes in health and safety requirements in relation to manual handling and moving. These directives stipulate that employers have a duty to ensure the safety of all employees involved in manual handling and moving activities. Employers are required to make a thorough assessment and implement measures to avoid risk. Where risk is unavoidable, they must take steps to minimise it. Employers also have a responsibility to make equipment and appropriate training available to all staff.

Employees' responsibilities

Employees have a responsibility to obey 'reasonable and lawful' instructions and to act with 'reasonable care and skill'. Thus, employees have a responsibility to attend training sessions provided by employers and to use equipment and handling aids according to the manufacturers' instructions. They also have a responsibility to inform the employers of any work situation that may require employees to work in a way that is dangerous to their health and safety. Although employers have a duty to perform risk assessments, employees equally have a responsibility to bring such situations to the employers' attention.

Safer-handling policies

Many hospitals and other institutions are working towards safer-handling or no-lifting policies. This requires the proper training and regular updating of all staff in the use of mechanical lifting equipment such as hoists, as well as sliding transfer aids and other equipment and techniques. Description of the techniques involved is beyond the scope of this book but there are a number of principles that may be applied to any handling situation.

Principles of safe handling

- Assess the situation. Is it necessary? Would the use of equipment be safer and more effective?
- Communicate clearly, so that all involved know what to expect.
- Avoid tensing the muscles.
- Adopt a stable stance – this usually means having your feet about a hip-width apart.
- Keep your knees 'soft' (slightly bent).
- Keep the load as close to your body as possible – avoid stretching.
- Keep your back in the natural alignment and avoid twisting or bending sideways.

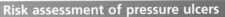

Principles

Pressure ulcers (also known as pressure sores and decubitus ulcers) have long been seen as costly both in terms of patient's health and in cost to the health service. In assessing patients' susceptibility to developing pressure ulcers a number of factors must be taken into consideration. These are generally grouped into two categories: external factors and internal factors.

External factors

- **Pressure** is the most important factor and occurs when the soft tissue of the body is compressed between a bony prominence and a hard surface.
- **Shear** occurs when the soft tissues and the skeleton move but the skin does not, e.g. sliding down the bed.
- **Friction** occurs when two surfaces rub together and the top layer of the skin is scraped off.

Internal factors

- Physical factors include the patients' general health, nutrition and hydration status, level of mobility, skin condition and restfulness/restlessness.
- Medical/surgical factors consider patients' cardiovascular system, continence status, medications, surgery, specific predisposing diseases and allergies.
- Psychological factors incorporate an assessment of patients' mental and emotional status that may affect sleep or motivation.
- Lifestyle factors include smoking and weight and build.
- Unchangeable factors are those such as age.

In order to provide consistent information and enable nurses to plan appropriate prevention strategies a number of assessment tools have been developed (e.g. Norton et al 1972, Waterlow 1995). These assessment tools differ but most consider the majority of factors outlined above. Clinical areas tend to use the one that is most suitable for their type of patients. What is important is that the nurse uses clinical judgement in conjunction with the chosen assessment tool as it is often the existence of a combination of factors that increases patients' susceptibility to pressure ulcer formation.

Assessing the patient

Assessment of the patient should address the following.

Physical factors

In combination with an assessment of patients' general health prior to admission to hospital, a thorough nutritional assessment should be undertaken (see page 98). This should include general dietary habits and pattern and fluid intake and hydration status. Current status in terms of whether the patient is nil-by-mouth, eating orally or being fed parenterally or enterally should be assessed. Patients' weight-to-height ratio should be calculated usually using the Body Mass Index Scale (BMI). Patients who have a poor diet lacking in vitamin C, proteins and minerals are more susceptible to pressure ulcer development.

Reduced nutritional status impairs the elasticity of the skin and skin that is dry (due to a poor or reduced fluid intake) is more susceptible to pressure damage.

When considering level of mobility, the nurse should consider activity level, presence of paralysis and restrictions to mobility (e.g. wound drains, intravenous infusions, traction or plaster) and whether these restrictions are temporary or permanent. Patients' general awareness, level of anxiety and the existence of pain should also be assessed.

Assessment of skin should consider whether it is healthy, papery, dry, clammy, sweaty or oedematous. Skin hydration should be noted and any evidence of previous ulceration, sores or broken skin or any pre-existing skin condition or discoloration. Assessing skin with a darker pigmentation needs to be undertaken very carefully as discoloration tends to be less noticeable. Patients' continence status should be considered as incontinence of urine and faeces can lead to skin maceration and constant washing can remove the natural oils thus drying the skin.

Medical/surgical history

Patients' previous medical or surgical history will indicate risk factors that impact on tissue perfusion and oxygenation of the tissues. Examples are diabetes, cardiovascular disease and anaemia. Any surgery including the length of time on the operating table, type of anaesthetic (e.g. epidural, spinal, general) should be noted. Medications should be considered, particularly noting antibiotics, steroids, sedatives, anti-inflammatory and cytotoxic drugs or insulin.

Psychological factors

Assessment of patients' emotional status (e.g. whether grieving or depressed) as this may affect their motivation.

Lifestyle factors

Whether a patient smokes should be noted as this may impact on respiratory function. When considering patients' weight and build, a note should be made of whether they are overweight or underweight.

Age

The age of the patient should be considered in conjunction with general health. Factors that impact on older patients (nutrition, skin elasticity, the presence of chronic illnesses) may not be significant for those who are younger.

Each of the factors above is allocated a score on the chosen assessment tool. The total indicates the level of risk, which in turn should indicate the nature of the prevention plan. However the allocation of scores for 'at-risk' conditions or behaviours is not consistent across the assessment tools. In some, a low total score indicates a high risk of pressure ulcer development, but in others, the opposite is true. There is considerable discussion in the literature as to the advantages and disadvantages of each tool. Currently there is no nationally agreed grading system.

The risk assessment should be documented in the nursing records along with preventative strategies. The assessment must be repeated at regular intervals as dictated by changes in the patient's condition, e.g. following surgery.

Principles

Prevention of pressure ulcers will not be achieved unless the predisposing factors are controlled or alleviated for each patient. Generic risk factors were previously identified but it is the particular combination of these in each patient that determines how high the risk is. Nevertheless there are general principles to follow when planning preventative strategies.

Regular repositioning

Frequent repositioning is essential whether the patient is in bed or in a chair. A useful yardstick is 2 hours, although this should be adjusted for the individual patient's need. Some patients, particularly those who are elderly, may need to be repositioned more regularly. The repositioning regimen must be rigorously implemented and in some cases can be supported by a 24-hour turning chart.

Careful positioning

Positioning when in bed and sitting in a chair is crucial. Where necessary patients should have the appropriate pressure-relieving mattress (Figure 13.1), although the effectiveness of the various types is the subject of much debate. The use of a pressure-relieving mattress does not remove the need to adjust the patient's position. The 30° tilt is thought to allow pressure to be tolerated for up to three times longer than over bony prominences (Gebhardt 2002). However, caution needs to be exercised in adopting this approach, as there is conflicting evidence regarding its clinical effectiveness. Bedclothes should be loose and sheets not wrinkled. Pillows can be used to support patients in the desired positions to prevent further deterioration brought about by incorrect positioning of limbs.

When seated in chairs patients should not be left for more than 2 hours regardless of the devices used. The chair must be of appropriate dimensions to promote good posture. There is little evidence that cushions are clinically effective for acutely ill patients but they may be of some benefit for those who are wheel-chair bound or have a chronic risk of developing pressure ulcers.

Exercise

Passive and active exercise is essential in maintaining and encouraging mobilisation and limiting the impact of some of the predisposing factors.

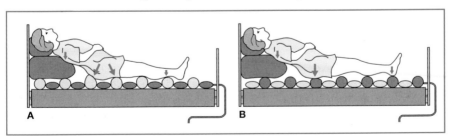

Figure 13.1 Alternating-pressure mattress

Safe moving and handling

When moving and handling patients, it is essential that appropriate manual handling equipment is used to prevent shear or friction. Positioning patients to prevent them sliding down the bed is important in preventing shear. The hospital backrest has been cited as the main culprit in encouraging sliding (Dealey 1999).

Nutrition and hydration

Consideration of patients' nutrition and hydration is important in order to maintain healthy skin and provide assistance with eating and drinking where necessary. Maintaining a food and fluid balance chart may be useful.

Skin care

Continuous assessment of the skin is vital. This can be undertaken when attending to the patient's hygiene needs. The skin should be kept clean and dry especially if the patient is incontinent, has a high temperature or is sweating excessively. Emollients in the bath or creams are useful for dry skin and a barrier cream for moist skin may be useful.

Preparation

Patient

- Patients who are immobile, undergoing surgery or have a predisposing factor are at risk of developing deep vein thrombosis (DVT).
- Dehydration and hypotension increase the risk.

Equipment/Environment

- Tape measure.
- Antiembolic stockings of appropriate size and length (calf or knee length).

Nurse

- The hands should be clean and an apron worn.

Procedure

1. Early mobilisation, if possible, reduces the risk of deep vein thrombosis (DVT).
2. Teach the patient foot and leg exercises before an operation or period of immobility and encourage exercises at least hourly **PFP1**. Position the patient's legs on the theatre table or in bed so as to prevent calf compression. Discourage the patient from crossing the legs in bed.
3. If the patient is unable to do foot and leg exercises, the nurse or physiotherapist should perform passive leg movements.
4. Deep breathing should be encouraged **PFP2**.
5. Observe the calves for swelling, heat and tenderness. If DVT is present, the calf may appear paler in colour than the calf of the other leg **PFP3**.
6. Measure the legs according to the manufacturer's instructions.
7. Fit the antiembolic stockings according to the manufacturer's instructions (Figure 13.2).
8. Subcutaneous heparin may be prescribed as a prophylactic measure.

Post procedure

Patient

- Encourage the patient to carry out leg movements and avoid activities that may increase the risk of DVT (e.g. crossing legs).

Equipment/Environment

- Remove anti-embolic stockings at least once daily, to inspect the skin and calves.
- Check frequently that the stockings are not wrinkled or rolled down.

Nurse

- Document the potential problem and nursing actions on the care plan.

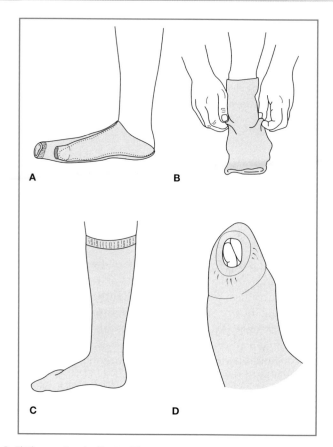

Figure 13.2 Fitting antiembolic stockings

Points for practice

1. Dorsiflexion (bending the feet up and down) and rotation of the feet encourages the lower leg muscles to 'pump' blood in the long saphenous vein, up towards the heart.

2. Movement of the diaphragm creates a negative pressure in the chest and inferior vena cava, which assists movement of blood towards the heart.

3. Evidence of DVT is most likely to occur from 48 hours post immobility.

Bibliography/Suggested reading

Moving and handling

Love C. Managing manual handling in clinical situations. *Nursing Times* 1995, **91**(26):38–39.

Love C. How to prevent injury caused by moving and handling. *Nursing Times* 1998, **94**(34):58–62.

National Back Pain Association & Royal College of Nursing. *The guide to the handling of patients*, revised 4th edn. London: NBPA; 1998.

Royal College of Nursing. *Code of practice for patient handling*. London: RCN; 1996.

Pressure ulcers

Cooper P, Gray D. Best practice statement for the prevention of pressure ulcers. *British Journal of Nursing* 2002 (Supplement) **11**(12): S39–S48.

Dealey C. *The care of wounds* 2nd ed. London: Blackwell, 1999

Department of Health. *Essence of care – patient-focussed benchmarking for health care practitioners*. London: DOH. 2001.

Gebhardt, K. Prevention of pressure ulcers – Part 1 Causes of pressure ulcers. *Nursing Times* 2002, **98**(11):41–44.

Gebhardt K. Prevention of pressure ulcers – Part 2 Patient assessment. *Nursing Times* 2002, **98**(12):39–42.

Gebhardt, K. Prevention of pressure ulcers – Part 3 Prevention strategies. *Nursing Times* 2002, **98**(13):37–40.

Morris L. Clinical practice benchmarking: implications for tissue viability. *British Journal of Nursing* 2002, **11**(12):Supplement 31–S36.

National Institute Clinical Excellence (NICE). *Pressure ulcer risk and prevention clinical guideline*. London: NICE; 2001.

Norton D, McLaren R, Exton-Smith A. *An investigation of geriatric nursing problems in hospital*. Edinburgh: Churchill Livingstone; 1972.

Royal College of Nursing. *Pressure ulcer risk assessment and prevention – clinical practice guidelines*. London: RCN, 2000.

Russell L. Pressure ulcer classification: the systems and the pitfalls. *British Journal of Nursing* 2002, **11**(12):Supplement 49–S59.

Waterlow J. Reliability of the Waterlow score. *Journal of Wound Care* 1995, **4**(10):474–475.

Deep Vein Thrombosis

Autar R. Nursing assessment of clients at risk of deep vein thrombosis: the Autar DVT scale. *Journal of Advanced Nursing* 1996, **23**(4):763–770.

Bright L, Georgi S. How to protect your patient from DVT. *American Journal of Nursing* 1994, **94**(12):28–32.

Geraghty S, Russell J, Gilbourne S, Young J. Deep vein thrombosis – aetiology and prevention. *Nursing Times* 2001, **97**(17):34–35.

Wallis M, Autar R. Deep vein thrombosis: clinical nursing management. *Nursing Standard* 2001, **15**(18):47–54.

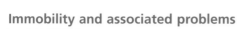
 Notes

Index

Index